Brain Allergies

Also by the authors:

Victory over Diabetes

Also by Dwight K. Kalita, Ph.D.:

Light Consciousness

A Physician's Handbook on Orthomolecluar Medicine
(with Roger J. William Ph.D.)

Nourishing Your Child
(with Ray Wunderlich, M.D.)

Brain Allergies

The Psychonutrient and Magnetic Connections

Second Edition

William H. Philpott, M.D.
and Dwight K. Kalita, Ph.D.

Foreword by Linus Pauling, Ph.D.

KEATS PUBLISHING
LOS ANGELES
NTC/Contemporary Publishing Group

This book is designed as a guide to patients undergoing professionally supervised, ecologic-orthomolecular diagnosis and treatment. The information also lends itself to self-help. For obvious reasons, its authors cannot take the medical or legal responsibility of having the contents herein considered as a prescription for anyone. Either you or the physician who examines and treats you must take the responsibility for the uses made of this book.

Library of Congress Cataloging-in-Publication Data

Philpott, William H., 1919–
Brain allergies: the psychonutrient and magnetic connections / William H. Philpott and Dwight K. Kalita ; foreword by Linus Pauling.—2nd ed.
p. cm.
Includes bibliographical references and index.
ISBN 0-658-00398-4
1. Food allergy—Complications. 2. Brain—Diseases—Nutritional aspects. 3. Mental illness—Nutritional aspects. 4. Diet therapy. 5. Orthomolecular therapy. I. Kalita, Dwight K. II. Title.

RC596 .P48 2000
616.97'5—dc21 99-055470

Published by Keats Publishing
A division of NTC/Contemporary Publishing Group, Inc.
4255 West Touhy Avenue, Lincolnwood (Chicago), Illinois 60712, U.S.A.

Printed in the United States of America

International Standard Book Number: 0-658-00398-4

6 7 8 9 0 DSH/DSH 0 1 0 9 8 7

To those patients who have sought so hard to find answers to their ecologic and nutritional problems. Those parents falsely accused of causing illnesses in their children that were in truth ecologic and nutritional in origin. Those researchers and clinicians swimming against the traditional tide of drug palliative, symptomatic relief while simultaneously exploring not only the mysteries of man maladaptively reacting to his physical environment but also the nutritional factors involved in all such reactions.

—William H. Philpott, M.D.

To my mother, Alice, the president of the Bio-Ecologic Research Center Inc., and my father, Arthur, who together as humanitarian medical researchers believe that the intensification of biochemical research and the practice of orthomolecular-ecologic medicine presently offer the greatest potential for the prevention and amelioration of degenerative diseases of all kinds. It is also dedicated to my wife, Bonnie, and my son Brian, whose love and tenderness daily create an uplifting source of inspiration.

—Dwight K. Kalita, Ph.D.

The Pioneers

We shall not travel by the road we make;
Ere day by day the sound of many feet
Is heard upon the stones that now we break,
We shall come to where the cross roads meet.

For us the heat by day, the cold by night,
The inch-slow progress, and the heavy load,
And death at last to close the long grim fight
With man and beast and stone; for them the road!

For them the shade of trees that now we plant,
For safe, smooth journey and the final goal,
Yea, birthright in the Land of Covenant—
For us day-labor, travail of the soul.

And yet the road is ours as never theirs!
Is not one joy on us alone bestowed?
For us the master: Joy, O Pioneers:
We shall not travel, but we make the Road.

—ANON.

CONTENTS

FOREWORD

One hundred years ago, it was rather generally accepted that mental disease is associated with an abnormality in the structure and composition of the brain. In the ninth edition of the *Encyclopedia Brittanica,* published in 1881, the statement was made that "It is universally accepted that the brain is the organ through which mental phenomena are manifested, and therefore that it is impossible to conceive of the existence of an insane mind in a healthy brain" (article on *Insanity*). There then followed a period, beginning during the early decades of the twentieth century and continuing to the present time, when the emphasis was on the psychological explanation of mental illness. During the last few years, another change has been taking place, in part, as a result of increased information about the structure of the brain and that its function is dependent upon its composition and structure. It is known that the presence in the brain of molecules of N, N-diethyl-D-lysergamide, mescaline, or other psychoactive substances is associated with profound psychic effects. As early as 1799, the English scientist Humphry Davy described various subjective reactions to the inhalation of the gas nitrous oxide. This gas and other anesthetic agents can, of course, produce general anesthesia, a pronounced change in the functioning of the brain.

The proper functioning of the brain is known to require the presence in the brain of molecules of many different substances. Mental disease, usually associated with physical disease, results from a low concentration of any one of a number of vitamins: thiamine (vitamin B_1), nicotinic acid or nicotinamide (B_3), pyridoxine (B_6), cobalamin (B_{12}), biotin, ascorbic acid (vitamin C), and folic acid. Other substances, which are not vitamins, also affect the functioning of the brain when a significant change in their concentration is achieved. Among these substances is glutamic acid, one of the amino acids that is present in proteins.

The concept that a change in behavior and in mental health can result from changing the concentrations of various substances that are normally present in the brain is an important one. This concept is the basis of *orthomolecular psychiatry*, a subject that is treated in considerable detail by Dr. William H. Philpott and Dr. Dwight K. Kalita in their book *Brain Allergies*. The other general concept, also a closely related one, is that of human ecology, the idea that substances in our environment can have a profound effect on mental health and behavior. These substances may be present in foods or in our natural environment, or they may be introduced into the environment as a result of our technological culture.

An allergy is the exaggerated reactivity of a living organism to a foreign substance that sometimes occurs following exposure to the substance, often even in a very small amount. Allergies are sometimes highly specific, caused by one substance and not by other closely related substances. Allergic reactions are believed to result from a combination of the molecules of the substance causing the allergy with substances characteristic of the body of the individual person. A considerable amount of information has been developed about the nature of the specific substances in a human being or animal that give rise to an allergic response. These specific substances are special protein molecules, usually called antibody molecules.

An exposure of a person to an allergen (a substance that can produce an allergic response) may sensitize the person in such a way that on later exposures to the allergen he responds in a characteristic way, often through abnormal behavior.

A vegetable or animal food eaten by a human being, unless it has been subjected to some unusual process of purification, consists of tens of thousands of substances of different kinds. The great majority of these substances might serve as antigens, sensitizing some people. Some allergies involve the brain in such a way that exposure to the particular allergen results in peculiarities of behavior.

In this book, *Brain Allergies*, Dr. Philpott and Dr. Kalita present a thorough discussion of this important field. I believe that many people will find it not only interesting but also valuable.

—LINUS PAULING
Linus Pauling Institute of Science and Medicine
Menlo Park, California

PREFACE

Hippocrates, the Father of Medicine, once said, "Leave your drugs in the chemist's pot if you can heal the patient with food." Since the first publication of this book in 1980, a significantly growing number of orthomolecular-ecologic psychiatrists have come to recognize the wisdom of Hippocrates. They now understand, for example, that drugs, which are foreign chemicals not normally found in the human body, radically alter man's biochemical/physiological environment. In doing so, these drug tranquilizers and antidepressants (e.g., phenothiazines, butyrophenones, SSRIs, etc.) control and/or suppress psychiatric symptoms. Unfortunately, the underlying metabolic disease process responsible for the mental symptoms in the first place usually remains unchecked.

In short, prescription drugs only provide symptomatic relief of mental and emotional illnesses. And because of this fact, they tend to mask the patient's fundamental metabolic problem but not eliminate it. In addition, they often create dangerous side effects that inadvertently add further complications to the underlying biochemical disease process.

Some of the serious side effects that are caused by the chronic use of symptom-suppressing tranquilizers include silent coronary death, tardive dyskinesia, Parkinsonism, and chemical dependencies. These drugs can also cause additional chemical addictions and even increase the possibility of developing clinical diabetes.

Needless to say, many orthomolecular-ecologic psychiatrists have become disillusioned with the symptom-suppressing results as well as with the serious side effects associated with the modern pharmacological incarceration of mentally ill patients. Consequently, these psychiatrists are now advocating a completely different type of medical treatment for the mentally ill. This alternative assumes that a healthy brain is fundamentally based on a healthy biochemical/nutritional, ecologic, and biomagnetic environment within each and every cell of the human body. In this regard, orthomolecular-ecologic psychiatrists are now turning their attention to a treatment modality that attempts to get at the etiology, or the root causes, of mental illness. Such an etiologically oriented treatment modality stresses the importance of the following three scientific procedures.

First, orthomolecular-ecologic psychiatrists firmly believe that foods, chemicals, and inhalants in the environment do indeed affect human behavior. In fact, they now understand that foods, chemicals, and inhalants can change the chemistry of our brain so dramatically that normal human behavior is radically altered. The end result of such a radical alteration of the brain's chemistry is called mental and emotional illness.

Such a dramatic change in human behavior occurs because of specific maladaptive allergic/addictive reactions to individually determined foods, chemicals, and inhalants encountered in everyday life. Orthomolecular-ecologic psychiatrists believe, therefore, that food, chemical, and inhalant immunologic allergies, addictions, and other nonimmunologic maladaptive reactions are the fundamental—indeed, the most significant—cause of minor as well as major mental and emotional illnesses. In short, these avant-garde physicians consider "brain allergies" to be the most important and promising area of research in the field of mental and emotional illnesses.

Orthomolecular-ecologic psychiatrists are thus centering their attention on the strict elimination of all symptom-producing substances—be they food, chemicals, or inhalants—as well as all addictions. This includes the implementation of the four-day diversified rotation diet, as well as the identification and avoidance of any foreign chemical stressors that may be present in the patient's environment.

These physicians consider the most important thing that can be done for the reversal of mental disorders is the identification and elimination of all food, chemical, and/or inhalant symptom-producing substances that are present in the patient's diet and/or environment. They believe this because they now know that the ecologic relationship between man and his food/chemical environment must be allergy-free and addiction-free in order to have healthy brain function. Accordingly, the proper testing and elimination of all offending food, chemical, and/or inhalant allergens is now the first and foremost goal of every orthomolecular-ecologic physician.

Years of deliberate food, chemical, and inhalant testing within the ranks of these physicians have provided convincing evidence that it is the stress of the *frequency of contact* that produces maladaptive, allergic/addictive reactions to foods, chemicals, and inhalants. This is true whether these reactions are immunoglobulin G (IgG) reactions or nonimmunological reactions. Generally speaking, the frequency of contact with an offending food, chemical, or inhalant needs to be more than two times per week.

As outlined in this book, the four-day diversified rotation diet, along with the strict avoidance of symptom-producing foods, chemicals, and inhalants, offers the best ecologically oriented treatment for moderate to severe mental and emotional symptoms. Such a rotation diet and strict avoidance procedure should be initiated simultaneously. A practical food rotation diet should be set up so as to avoid any food eaten as frequently as two times a week or more. These frequently eaten foods should be avoided for three months. After this period, the foods left out of the diet can be introduced back into the four-day diversified rotation diet.

Many patients have no symptoms once these foods are reintroduced. However, gluten-containing wheat, rye, oats, or barley, as well as dairy foods, corn products, individually determined foods, and many hydrocarbon-based chemicals and/or inhalants sometimes can never be reintroduced into the patient's diet and/or living environment. In such cases, these allergy-producing substances must be avoided permanently.

After years of observing maladaptive mental reactions to foods, most orthomolecular-ecologic psychiatrists would agree that gluten is the most frequent and severe symptom reactor of all foods. As a result, gluten is the most likely food substance to evoke physical as well as mental symptoms. However, it is important to keep in mind that many other foods, chemicals, and inhalants can also cause severe maladaptive reactions.

Common physical reactions to gluten include gastrointestinal problems, such as celiac disease, Crohn's disease (gluten enteropathy), jerking muscles (Tourette's syndrome), and headache. Emotional and mental symptoms caused by reactions to gluten range from mild tension, anxiety, phobias, depression, obsessions, compulsion, and so forth to severe psychotic depression, hallucinations, and delusions.

In addition to being the most reactive food substance in terms of immunologic and nonimmunologic maladaptive reactions, gluten is the most addictive of all food substances. Gluten is split in half during the first stage of digestion, which occurs in the stomach by a combination of hydrochloric acid with the enzyme pepsin. This splitting of gluten produces an active narcotic called *exorphin*. This narcotic becomes addictive when it is absorbed through the small intestine without further digestion by pancreatic enzymes, sodium, and potassium bicarbonate.

Orthomolecular-ecologic psychiatrists are now using a second major etiologically based treatment modality for the mentally ill. They insist, for example, on the regulation of optimum dietary nutrition in the treatment of all their patients. *Orthomolecular-ecologic psychiatrists suggest that the treatment of mental diseases should include varying the concentration of "right molecules"—that is, vitamins, minerals, trace elements, essential fatty acids, enzymes, amino acids, and hormones—that normally occur in the human body*. This right molecule, or orthomolecular, approach to medicine includes the compensation for, as well as the correction of, any nutritional deficiencies that might be present in their patients.

The list of nutritional substances needed by the human body for optimum mental as well as physical health includes the following:

Essential Fatty Acids	Linoleic Acid Linolenic Acid	***Minerals***	Calcium Chlorine Chromium Cobalt Copper Fluorine Iodine Iron Magnesium Manganese Molybdenum Nickel Phosphorus Potassium Selenium Silicon Sodium Strontium Sulphur Vanadium Zinc
Amino Acids	Arginine (essential for children) Histidine (essential for children) Isoleucine Leucine Lysine Methionine Phenylalanine Threonine Tryptophan Valine		
Vitamins	Biotin (B_7) Cobalamin (B_{12}) Folic Acid (B_9) Niacin (B_3) Pantothenic Acid (B_5) Pyridoxine (B_6) Riboflavin (B_2) Thiamine (B_1) Vitamin A Vitamin C Vitamin D Vitamin E Vitamin K		

Orthomolecular-ecologic psychiatrists seek to regulate all of these nutritional chemical substances that are already present in the human body at birth. Instead of relying only on chemical substances that are not normally found in the human body (i.e., drugs), orthomolecular-ecologic psychiatrists are now seeing extremely positive results when their patients are treated at the cellular level with biological weapons (i.e., nutrients) that nature has provided in her own structure of defense since the beginning of life.

Listed below is a partial description of nutritional supplements found to be effective in treating maladaptive mental reactions to foods, chemicals, and inhalants. Vitamin C is best taken as ascorbates of calcium, magnesium, zinc, selenium, manganese, and copper. Antioxidants such as vitamin E, beta-carotene, and vitamin A should be given according to individual need. It is also recommended that there be a periodic laboratory assessment of each individual's nutritional state. This is especially true when determining amino acid and/or mineral nutritional needs.

Nutritional Supplement	***Dosage***
Vitamin C as ascorbates	5–12 g/day
Magnesium	250–500 mg/day
Zinc	15–30 mg/day
Niacin	500–3,000 mg/day
Vitamin B_6	25–100 mg/day
Vitamin B_{12}	1,000 mg/day
Amino acids	
cystine	500 mg
taurine	500 mg
Proteolytic enzymes	——
Essential fatty acids	
(fish oils, primrose oil, flaxseed oil, etc.)	——

Such a medically informed regulation of dietary nutritional substances is extremely important to every patient's optimum mental health. If cell deficiencies of any of the above nutrients occur, then the concentration of these nutrients, which are needed for optimum mental health, must be altered according to the individual patient's unique needs. Moreover, this nutritional alteration includes the elimination of all toxic minerals such as lead, mercury, arsenic, cadmium, and the like from the patient's body.

We can discover one example of the vast number of nutritional deficiencies that currently exist in the average American diet by examining the area of essential fatty acids (EFAs). If researchers are correct, approximately 80 percent of our population are deficient in EFAs. These EFAs include linoleic acid and linolenic acid. These important human nutrients are needed biochemically by both our bodies and our brains and are available to us only from our diet. Grapeseed oil, borage oil, flaxseed oil, and so forth are all good sources of EFAs.

In regard to the essential nature of EFAs, the hormonelike substances known as prostaglandins require EFAs for their proper synthesis. Prostaglandins, as researchers have now discovered, play an important role in reducing various types of inflammatory reactions, be they allergic or other. If the American public is deficient in EFAs, then many of us may lack one of nature's most important means—namely, prostaglandins—of controlling inflammatory allergic reactions, be they in the brain or some other part of the body.

Even more disturbing is the fact that multiple nutrient deficiencies are occurring throughout a growing number of people in our country. Luckily, these nutrient deficiencies are treatable if they are properly diagnosed. Since 1980, many developments have improved the diagnostic process. Improved techniques have developed for assessing vitamins, minerals, amino acids, and EFAs. IgG food testing has replaced cytotoxic testing. Other improvements have been developed in the areas of examining viral and fungal states and monitoring oxidative enzyme function. Hair testing for minerals has been replaced by mineral assessment of whole blood and red blood cells. Hair testing is now used primarily for determining the levels of toxic minerals.

In addition, antibody studies for Epstein-Barr virus, cytomegalovirus, and human herpes virus #6 are now a significant aspect of every differential diagnosis. The importance of testing for isolatable neurotrophic and lymphotrophic viruses becomes more obvious when one understands that there is a common starting point for all the varying degrees of organic brain disorders (e.g., hyperkinesis, manic depressive disorders, dyslexia, autism, schizophrenia, etc.). This common denominator in all these organic brain disorders is a viral infection from the herpes family of lymphotrophic viruses: Epstein-Barr virus, cytomegalovirus, and human herpes virus #6.

The infection has its inception in early childhood before the brain has reached its maturity in late adolescence. There is literally a chronic, smoldering, viral encephalitis progressively injuring the brain, especially in the areas that deal with emotion, judgment, and perception. The infection is progressive and can manifest itself as a minor brain disorder in childhood and end up in late adolescence or the early twenties as a major psychosis. Antibody studies over a number of years have revealed that these types of viral infections in the brain are chronic and fluctuating.

As a result of the chronic stress of these previously undetected viral infections, there develops a state of maladaptive allergic reactions to foods, chemicals, and/or inhalants that further exacerbates the mental symptoms. In addition, severe nutritional and immunological deficiencies also develop in this vicious circle of biochemical cerebral deterioration. It is precisely at this stage of deterioration that the orthomolecular-ecologic psychiatrist must step in and reverse the nutritionally deficient, maladaptive allergic reactions that occur in most, if not all, chronic and organically based mental illnesses.

In addition to the ecologic and orthomolecular treatment modalities previously discussed, *the orthomolecular-ecologic psychiatrist now has a new and very promising third etiologically based weapon to use in the battle against mental and emotional illness: biomagnetic therapy.*

In order to introduce this exciting new biomagnetic treatment modality, let us first update a case history that was reported in *Brain Allergies* when it was first published almost twenty years ago (see page 20). It involves a man named Karl who was psychotic. He had the delusion that he was Jesus Christ. Karl, as it turned out, was extremely allergic to certain foods as well as petrochemical hydrocarbons. Commonly experienced items that contain petrochemical hydrocarbons include candles, waxes, sprays, fresheners, perfumes, certified food coloring, exhaust fumes, and pesticides.

Karl's illness became manifest when he sprayed an apple orchard with a specific pesticide. He also had an apple warehouse, which was an enclosed cooler. One day he became so weak that he fell off the forklift. He was taken to the emergency room of a local hospital where he was diagnosed to be psychotic. He became my patient shortly thereafter. I found him not only reactive to an assortment of petrochemical hydrocarbons but also to a number of foods.

By avoiding the foods that Karl frequently used, and by avoiding exposure to chemicals in his home and work environment, he became mentally clear within a period of five days. Upon being exposed to petrochemical hydrocarbons such as an extract of car exhaust or pesticides, he immediately became delusional, thinking again that he was Jesus Christ.

The interesting point about Karl is that after identifying and strictly avoiding specific foods and chemicals, as well as treating his nutritional deficiencies, he was sane for nineteen years. Recently, however, he suddenly became psychotic again when his neighbor tarred his roof with a hot, smelly tar. This time he was treated with two neodymium disc magnets. These relatively inexpensive magnets were placed bitemporally on his head. Within ten to fifteen minutes of the magnet therapy, his delusional symptoms were completely gone. Karl was sane again!

Karl also discovered that he could significantly reduce his chances of recurring symptoms by sleeping on a magnetic bed pad and with magnets at the crown of his head. Quite understandably, he keeps the neodymium disc magnets with him at all times. If he does by chance have exposure to any petrochemical hydrocarbons, he places the magnets bitemporally, and all his mental symptoms are relieved shortly thereafter. Fortunately, he does not have to use any tranquilizers or antidepressants.

Tim is another patient who had dramatic results with magnetic therapy. At age five, he was correctly diagnosed by a children's hospital as autistic. As both his parents were medical doctors, he was given every therapeutic, medical, and educational opportunity available. At age seventeen, he became my patient. He was obviously schizophrenic and could only speak in grunts accompanied by bizarre facial and arm movements. Much of the time, even his mother could not understand anything that he was attempting to say.

Episodically, Tim experienced periods of saying the word "circle" at three-second intervals. When the negative (south-seeking) pole of the 4-inch by 6-inch by ½-inch magnet was placed on the back of his head and upper neck, he would stop his compulsive, repetitive verbalization. Deliberate food testing demonstrated that any gluten-bearing foods would evoke this same symptom immediately. His psychosis cleared by the fifth day of his avoidance of commonly eaten foods and all chemicals. When his psychotic symptom-evoking foods, which had been determined by deliberate food tests of single foods, were returned to his four-day diversified rotation diet after three months of strict avoidance, they no longer produced any symptoms.

With behavioral training and the use of temporally placed magnets, he was taught to speak clearly without his former bizarre facial and arm gesturing. He was also diagnosed to be cystine- and taurine-deficient and was supplemented with these two amino acids accordingly. Eventually, he was taught to drive a car and attended a university as a special student in the art department. He was able to maintain his own apartment and even prepare his own food for his four-day diversified rotation diet.

After discovering the combined positive results of orthomolecular-ecologic-biomagnetic therapy, Tim, an autistic at age five and a schizophrenic as an adolescent, has now become a socially and economically functional part of our society.

The physicist Albert Roy Davis's observations concerning the opposite biological response to opposite magnetic poles set the stage for understanding the therapeutic powers of magnets. It is now known, for example, that magnetism functions at the atomic level with the movement of electrons. The positive magnetic field (north-seeking pole) spins electrons clockwise, while the negative magnetic field (south-seeking pole) spins electrons counterclockwise. When the human body is exposed to these two magnetic fields, the opposite electron spins from the opposite magnetic fields provide predictable and opposite biological responses within each cell of the human body.

More specifically, the positive magnetic field is the signal of stress injury. In terms of neuronal response, the positive magnetic field produces an exciting effect within the cells of the human body. When this exciting effect is sufficiently high—for example, when sun flares occur—it can precipitate psychosis in those so biologically predisposed. The strength of any magnetic field is quantified as its *gauss strength*. The higher the gauss strength, the higher the excitement. A positive magnetic field of sufficiently high gauss strength can even evoke seizures in those so predisposed.

The negative magnetic field, on the other hand, governs healing and normalization of biological functions. The negative magnetic field is neuron-calming and encourages rest, relaxation, sleep, and healing. When it is sufficiently high in gauss strength, it can even produce general anesthesia. In addition, the higher the gauss of the negative magnetic field, the slower the brain-pulsing on an EEG.

In recent years, this information set the stage in our understanding of how a negative magnetic field controls neuronal excitement in neurosis, psychosis, seizures, addictions, brain allergies, addictive withdrawals, and movement disorders. It also offered us a more solid foundation upon which to build our understanding of precisely how the negative magnetic field alters human biological responses.

In particular, acid hypoxia is present during all acute allergic reactions to foods, chemicals, or inhalants. Moreover, when a patient comes in contact with a food, chemical, or inhalant to which he is maladaptively reactive, the body produces dangerous, symptom-producing free radicals such as hydrogen peroxide, hydroxyl radicals, acids, alcohols, and aldehydes. All of these harmful by-products of allergic maladaptive reactions thrive in an acid state.

Furthermore, free radicals produce inflammation and/or swelling within each cell that is affected by the maladaptive reaction. Free-radical damage and inflammation continue to influence the cells in this maladaptive acid state. This entire biochemical process further produces a deficiency of oxygen within the damaged cells. Needless to say, any oxygen-deficient state is extremely harmful to human cells, be these cells in the body or in the brain.

When the cells within the brain malfunction in the previously described fashion, depression, hallucinations, delusions, obsessive/compulsiveness, and so forth are the likely results. The correction of these symptoms requires an immediate normalization of the pH back to its alkaline state. This, in turn, releases oxygen from its bound state in the free radicals, and healing begins to occur.

We now understand that the negative magnetic field evokes a biological response of alkaline-hyperoxia. In other words, the negative magnetic field immediately reverses any maladaptive acid state within the cells of the human body back to an alkaline state. It does so by producing a biological response of activating, normalizing, and maintaining the bicarbonate buffer system. It also serves as the energy activator of the oxidoreductase enzymes. These unique enzymes release oxygen from its bound state in free radicals, organic peroxides, and so forth back to molecular oxygen.

The negative magnetic field reduces all types of inflammation and maladaptive reactions, be these reactions physiological or mental in nature. The negative magnetic field does so because it first activates oxidoreductase enzymes. These enzymes then enzymatically process free radicals, peroxides, acids, alcohols, and aldehydes. This biochemical reaction results in the release of molecular oxygen from its bound state in these substances. Hence, the healing powers of molecular oxygen as well as alkaline-hyperoxia occur!

This biochemical process is important to understand because it offers an insight as to why the negative magnetic field so quickly reverses maladaptive reactions. It explains why any particular symptom can be eliminated within ten minutes or so, whether this symptom is an inflammatory pain or maladaptive reaction, by placing a sufficiently high-gauss negative magnet over the affected area.

The explanation is, of course, that the human body's metabolism functions optimally only with the constant maintenance of alkaline-hyperoxia at all levels (i.e., cellular, tissue, organ, and systemic). Acute symptom-producing maladaptive reactions are locally acid-hypoxic in the cells and tissues where symptoms occur. The negative field of a magnet immediately alkalinizes as well as oxygenates the acid-hypoxic cells, tissues, and organs being treated. And the fact is no inflammatory or maladaptive reaction can occur when there is a sufficient supply of oxygen and alkalinity.

Regarding the immediate healing powers of biomagnetic energy, it has been observed that when a person has an insect bee sting and places a negative magnetic field of sufficient gauss strength over the sting area, no swelling occurs. There is literally no inflammatory reaction. It is also gratifying to observe that a superficial burn, which blanches the skin and causes immediate pain, is immediately relieved when the burn victim places a negative magnetic field over the burn.

However, the most important value of magnetic therapy involves mental and emotional disorders. Anxiety, depression, phobias, obsessive/compulsiveness, delusions, hallucinations, and psychotic depression have all been successfully treated with magnetic therapy. The negative magnetic field has the capacity to reduce minor emotional responses, maladaptive allergic reactions, and addictions, as well as major mental disorder responses, including seizures.

Obviously, any successful magnetic-therapy program requires a magnet of appropriate gauss strength and the appropriate placement of the magnet to achieve the desired goals. Fortunately, the negative magnetic field does not raise endorphins beyond the normal range and is therefore not addictive. In addition, there are no limits to the duration of exposure. Most symptoms are relieved within ten minutes, although some occasionally require as much time as thirty minutes. The symptoms usually stay away for an extended period, and the magnetic field application can be repeated as often as necessary.

Regarding the proper placement of magnets, the negative magnetic field of a permanent static field magnet should be placed directly over the affected area. The higher the gauss strength, the more efficient the treatment. The magnets used are flat-surfaced magnets with poles on opposite sides of the flat surfaces.

For the treatment of major mental disorders, disc magnets are often placed bitemporally, on the midforehead and left temporal, or left temporal and occipital, depending on the mental symptoms being treated. Patients should also use magnetic mattress pads and ceramic block magnets in a carrier up against the headboard while sleeping in bed.

For the specifics of such treatment procedures of the mentally ill, patients should consult a physician who has had clinical experience in the areas of magnetic therapy and mental illness. The manufacturer's gauss strength of each magnet is listed in the table below. The patient actually receives one-third of the manufacturer's gauss rating.

Magnet	***Gauss Strength***
1½" x ½" ceramic disc magnets	3,950 gauss strength
1" x ¼" super neodymium disc magnets	12,300 gauss strength
1 ⅞" x ⅞" x ⅜" ceramic miniblock magnets	3,950 gauss strength
4" x 6" x ½" ceramic block magnet with Velcro	3,950 gauss strength
4" x 6" x 1" ceramic block magnets	3,950 gauss strength

The treatment of the mentally and emotionally ill by such noninjurious methods as avoidance of maladaptive reactions to foods, chemicals, and inhalants; the four-day diversified rotation diet; appropriate nutritional testing and treatment; and magnetic therapy offers the greatest hope for the future. Clearly, these methods require a new set of tests and observations that today are not familiar even to specialists in highly trained areas of medicine. In particular, they require a new, expanded, and more specialized set of information, skills, tests, and orientation not normally taught in today's medical schools.

Unfortunately, standard textbooks in neurology and psychiatry make no mention of maladaptive reactions to foods, chemicals, and inhalants as precipitating causes of mental and emotional illnesses. Neither are neurologists and psychiatrists taught a systematic method of examining for maladaptive reactions. To remedy this shortcoming, the specialties of neurology and psychiatry need to add the skills of optimum nutritional management; diagnosis and therapeutic management of immunologic and nonimmunologic maladaptive symptom-producing reactions to foods, chemicals, and inhalants; and magnetic therapy. Such a program of treatment would not only dispense with the often injurious side effects of tranquilizers, antidepressants, and other medications, but it would also provide enormous economic savings to those who are chronically ill.

When treating a specific and serious mental and/or emotional illness, one should of course seek the advice of a trained orthomolecular-ecologic psychiatrist who has had experience in the field of magnetic therapy. Magnetic therapy, combined with the previously described orthomolecular and ecologic treatment modalities, can successfully replace tranquilizers, antidepressants, and electroconvulsive treatment, and do so without side effects. As a psychiatrist, I am experienced in the use of tranquilizers and antidepressants and have administered an excess of 70,000 electroconvulsive treatments. Based on this experience, I believe that the orthomolecular-ecologic-biomagnetic therapy program is superior to all of the more traditional methods of treating emotional and mental illness.

—William H. Philpott, M.D., and Dwight K. Kalita, Ph.D.

ACKNOWLEDGMENTS

S. Klotz, M.D., allergist, deserves special mention for suggesting in 1970 that there might be profit in examining central nervous system maladaptive reactions to foods, chemicals, and inhalants in emotional and behavioral disorders. He deserves special credit for a positive double-blind study of provocative testing of allergies, which provided the courage to proceed with further testing.

Marshall Mandell, M.D., allergist, has been most important in guiding the application of provocative testing in emotionally ill patients. His valuable guidance laid the foundation upon which was built a systematic evaluation of ecologic mental illness. The double-blind study of provocative testing made by Dr. Mandell and David King, Ph.D., has helped establish the scientific validity of this approach.

Theron G. Randolph, M.D., allergist, through his meticulous observations and remarkable ability of correlating information, laid the foundation for understanding the value and uses of provocative testing, understanding the role of addiction in the degenerative disease process, and establishing the fact of ecologic mental illness.

Martin Rubin, Ph.D., biochemist, deserves special credit for the initial guidance in and continued support of the laboratory role in a search for biological factors in mental illness. His recommendation of using stress type testing to determine vitamin deficiencies and metabolic disorders led to the use of provocative testing of reactive substances as the stressors in testing for the biology of these disorders.

Jay Shurley, M.D., psychiatrist, deserves special mention for the positive Task Force Report on "Relating Environment to Mental Health and Illness: The Eco-Psychiatry Data Base."

Khaja Khaleeluddin, Ph.D., chemist, has been most helpful in deciphering the meaning of laboratory findings. He did much to help discover the evidence of B_6 utilization disorder and the significance of disordered methionine metabolism.

Chapter 1

Nutrient Therapy

Two thousand five hundred years ago, Hippocrates, the "Father of Medicine," said to his students, "Let thy food be thy medicine and thy medicine be thy food." Moses Maimonides, the great twelfth-century physician, repeated the Hippocratic sentiment when he said, "No illness which can be treated by diet should be treated by any other means." In essence, Hippocrates and Maimonides were insisting that their students practice *nutrient therapy.* This type of medical therapy is being used by physicians today, though only by a minority. There is, however, a rapidly developing rebirth of interest in this unique orientation, and physicians all around the world are beginning to look more closely at the wisdom of the "Father of Medicine."

Today, nutrient therapy is basically composed of two medical disciplines: orthomolecular medicine and human ecology. The first term was coined in 1968 by Linus Pauling, Ph.D., twice a Nobel Prize winner. "Orthomolecular" is, literally, "pertaining to the right molecule." Orthomolecular physicians believe that the treatment of infectious and degenerative diseases should be a matter of varying the concentration of "right molecules" (i.e., vitamins, minerals, trace elements, amino acids, enzymes, hormones, etc.) which are normally present in the human body. This belief is based on the idea that the nutritional microenvironment of every cell in our body is extremely important to our optimum health, and deficiencies in this environment constitute the major cause of disease. If cell deficiencies do develop, the concentration of the nutrients needed for optimum health must be altered according to individual needs. The assumption here is that if each biochemically individual cell of our bodies is provided with the optimum nutrients necessary for its proper and healthy functioning, then the internal environment will be at its optimum for the individual, and chronic degenerative diseases will eventually be controlled.

The list of necessary nutrients is the same for every human being, but the relative amounts needed by each individual are as distinctively different as fingerprints. Why is this? Because the kind of food you eat, the physical, mental, and emotional stress you experience, the environment in which you live and work, your unique, individually determined biochemical heredity pattern, the type of soil in which your food is grown, the type of water you drink, the amount of exercise you have, all add up to determine the fact that your body is not a conglomeration of cells needing a "one for all and all for one" minimum daily requirement. You are a unique individual with unique biochemical needs. If your body cells are ailing, as they do in any form of human disease, the chances are good that it is because they are not being adequately provided with the optimum nutrients they need to sustain and propagate healthy human tissues, organs, and life in general. In other words, cellular health is not based on a *minimum daily requirement* but on an *optimum daily need* determined by your own biochemical uniqueness. This is precisely where orthomolecular medicine comes to the front lines in the battle against disease. Many medical men, including psychiatrists, are beginning to observe positive clinical results when their patients are treated at the cellular level with biological weapons—nutrients—nature has provided in her own structure of defense since the beginning of life. By contrast, *toximolecular* medicine, a type of therapy used by the majority of physicians in our country for only the past forty years, is the administration of drugs at sublethal levels. Drugs, of course, are alien chemicals that are not normally present in the cellular environment of the human body. They radically alter man's biochemical-physiological internal environment and often occasion very severe and dangerous side effects. Needless to say, drugs do not halt or prevent the disease process, especially degenerative disease; at best they offer symptomatic relief, while the fundamental, underlying disease process continues uninterrupted.

"The basic fault of these weapons [drugs]," writes Roger J. Williams, Ph.D., "is that they have no known connection with the disease process itself. . . . Drugs are wholly unlike nature's weapons. . . . They tend to mask the difficulty, not eliminate it. They contaminate the internal environment [with side effects], create dependence on the part of the patient, and often complicate the physician's job by erasing valuable clues as to the real source of the trouble."[1]

A tragic example of this statement is provided by Peter, a forty-five-year-old schizophrenic, who took Thorazine® (a phenothiazine tranquilizer) for five years. One year after first taking Thorazine, he began to have a masklike face and to walk stiffly without swinging his arms. He was placed on an antiparkinsonian medication and continued on Thorazine because as soon as it was stopped he became psychotic. Now he is like a shaking zombie: not swinging his arms and continuing to tremor in both arms and legs. Today, the symptoms continue even when the Thorazine is removed. Peter, in short, has permanent parkinsonism caused by Thorazine.

Sally, another tragic example, is twenty-five years old, and for three years has been on the butyrophenone tranquilizer Haldol®. Her head jerks from side to side, and her tongue moves in her mouth continuously. The symptoms continue even though the tranquilizer has been discontinued. She has tardive dyskinesia caused by Haldol.

The incidence of acute evoked parkinsonism and tardive dyskinesia with the use of phenothiazines and butyrophenones is beginning to alarm the medical profession.[2] The evidence of chronicity of these iatrogenic—physician-induced—illnesses further increases the concern. The United States Public Health Department is warning doctors not to use these drugs if side effects occur or to be prepared to justify their continued use in reacting patients. A detailed discussion of the nature and specific causes of some drug-induced illnesses, and methods by which some have been successfully treated, is given in the appendix.

Furthermore, physicians and patients alike have a right to be alarmed at the growing list of evidences of adverse and even fatal reactions to the chronic use of phenothiazines. Consider such side effects as allergic skin reactions, allergic bone marrow reactions producing agranulocytosis, hepatitis, and the deterioration of the conduction system of the heart. Silent coronary death due to a phenothiazine-induced (Stelazine®, Thorazine, and the like) deterioration of the heart's conduction system may be one of the most serious threats of prolonged drug use. I was personally alerted to, and alarmed by, this possibility when a patient died a silent coronary death. Autopsy revealed her heart's conduction system to be deteriorated in a manner that has been associated with chronic phenothiazine use, a drug she had been on for five years. It has been estimated that these silent coronary deaths with demonstrable deteriorated heart conduction systems in older chronic phenothiazine-tranquilized patients may be occurring at the approximate rate of one in a thousand patients. Even without absolute proof of the accuracy of either the association or the frequency of these silent coronaries in chronic tranquilized patients, it remains a subject to be investigated.

Using an injectible phenothiazine tranquilizer in a controlled study on rats, one researcher demonstrated a 20 percent loss of brain cells in the corpus stratum. This experiment shows the significance of a phenothiazine-producing destructive reaction in the brain area responsible for parkinsonism and tardive dyskinesia. Microscopic evidence proves that this occurs in rats; clinical evidence indicates that it occurs in humans. Therefore, doctors are shouldering a lot of responsibilities when using phenothiazines and butyrophenones for their patients. Psychiatrists, in particular, have been fooled by the short-term values of symptom reduction in patients given major tranquilizers; however, they are awakening to the fact that they are on the horns of a dilemma in which the side effects of phenothiazines and butyrophenones are becoming as serious as the original illness itself. That is, the tranquilized patient is basically still sick and loaded with symptoms, inefficient, nonproductive, and dependent upon others for survival; now, however, he is under the threat of developing a chronic illness or even of dying. "There are too many closed doors," writes then Senator Harold E. Hughes, "too many closed minds in our traditional approach to health care. We need the courage and the sense to strike out in new directions where the old ways have failed."[3]

After reflecting on the drug situation as it really is, it is easy to see why orthomolecular physicians believe, as Hippocrates observed, that nature's biological nutrients, a defense system used for millions of years in the battle against all forms of disease, are far more reliable and more time-proven than the relatively recent drug-therapy fads that have swept the modern world. This is particularly true in our battle against the degenerative diseases. It is unfortunately true that a few years ago, the population in one year swallowed 1,542,000 pounds of tranquilizers, 836,000 pounds of barbiturates, and 4,037,000 pounds of penicillin; yet 93 million of 213 million people in the United States (almost half the population!) suffer from some form of degenerative disease. These statistics get worse every year. Obviously, symptomatic drug therapy is not getting at the heart of the nation's health problems.

The other equally important side of nutrient therapy is called human ecology, which scientifically examines man's environment in order to discover sources of environmentally produced illness. The word *environment* is here used in a very broad sense: It includes every chemical and food with which a person may come in contact. According to this concept, the field of allergies is much larger than traditional immunologists have claimed. There are many maladaptive, allergic-like reactions, including central-nervous-system reactions, which do not manifest antibody formation and, therefore, do not fit the immunologist's narrow definition of allergy.

Clinical ecology is a more inclusive term and includes all maladaptive reactions—physical, mental, emotional, or otherwise—occurring on exposure to any substance—a food, chemical, or pollutant. As a group of susceptible patients were subjected to ecologically oriented testing methods, evaluations, and diagnosis, the following progressive levels of reactions were recorded: acute localized physical effects (rhinitis, bronchitis, asthma, eczema, and gastrointestinal and other allergies); acute systemic effects (headache, fatigue, myalgia, arthralgia, neuralgia, and other generalized physical syndromes); and acute mental effects (confusion, depression, delusions, hallucinations, and other advanced cerebral and behavioral abnormalities). When these chronic symptoms were studied by means of comprehensive environmental control, clinically induced reexposures to the incriminating substances gave predictable results. It was during the course of these clinical experiences that the dominant role of chemical and food allergies in producing "ecologic" physical and mental illnesses became apparent. Physicians discovered that they were indeed dealing with the etiology—the root causes—of many of their patients' illnesses.

But why are the majority of physicians in our country oriented toward the toximolecular approach in medicine? An answer comes in part from the hearing before the Select Committee on Nutrition and Human Needs of the United States Senate, held on June 22, 1977:

> *Senator George McGovern:* Achieving recognition of the relationship between nutrition and [mental] health is still very much a struggle. Established scientific thinking remains weighted against those few scientists and practitioners who are striving to understand the complex links between the food we consume and how we think and behave as individuals. For example, the newly appointed Mental Health Commission has no member with experience in this vital area. I find this oversight both surprising and distressing. . . . If further research is undertaken along a nutritional line, we could find that a significant number of mental health problems could be cured or prevented by better nutrition. . . .

> *Senator McGovern to Mike Lesser, M.D.:* You referred to the fact that some 50 percent of our hospitals' beds are filled with individuals

> suffering from schizophrenia. With the methods we are not using, are we not simply adding to the burden of the hospitals and perpetuating a system of therapy [i.e., toximolecular] that may help the drug industry but really is not dealing with the basic problem?
>
> *Dr. Lesser:* I believe we are. I believe that is the situation. We are just providing symptomatic relief and control at this moment and not getting at the basic cause. Tranquilizers came out in the fifties. Fortunately or unfortunately, for the treatment of mental illness, tranquilizers are drugs, and therefore patentable substances. In other words, a pharmaceutical house can receive an exclusive monopoly to produce that particular substance for, I believe, ten years. This allows the company to make money off of that drug. This money pays for research into further use of drugs. It also pays to hire detail men to visit physicians who are treating patients, and every physician in this country is currently visited by detail men who tell him about the latest drug discoveries. . . . It also pays for the testing necessary in order to receive federal government approval to use those drugs. . . . Vitamins [all nutrients] are not patentable substances. Nutrients are available in nature and no one can patent them.
>
> *Senator Schweiker:* The FDA tried to ban them a year and a half ago. We had to fight that.
>
> *Dr. Lesser:* The physicians in medical school are taught to use drugs, not nutrients. Hours are spent teaching physicians how to prescribe various drugs to treat disease.[4]

Indeed, nutrient therapy is more effective than toximolecular therapy because it recognizes that a healthy body is based on healthy cells. And all cells depend for their very existence on vitamins, minerals, trace elements, amino acids, enzymes, and so on—the nutrients used by orthomolecular-ecological physicians. The simple truth is that our country needs physicians who are interested in curing and preventing the causes of disease rather than merely in symptomatic treatment and relief. If we fail at this task, then the medical field will not be the third largest industry in our country as it is today, but the largest. If this tragedy occurs, and statistical analysis suggests it well might be in the next decade, then it will take the entire Gross National Product to support its existence! Nutrient therapy, on the other hand, is a safe, economical, prevention-oriented, and, as we shall see, effective alternative to our current medical crisis.

Chapter 2

From a Philospher-Psychiatrist to a True Scientist

One must be taught to suspect, for if one does not suspect, he does not test, and if he does not test, he does not know.[5]

—H. J. RINKEL

In 1950, I along with a dozen other senior medical students attended a presentation by Alfred Rouse, M.D., an allergist. He presented the case of a woman who became anxious when given a specific food. Then he asked, "What is the diagnosis?" I had taken medicine with the express purpose of becoming a psychiatrist and prided myself on having learned psychiatric diagnosis. Drawing on the methods I had been taught, I gave the answer: anxiety neurosis. Dr. Rouse rejected this and to my surprise maintained almost pleadingly that an allergic reaction was involved. All I obtained from this experience at the time was that he did not appreciate my diagnostic ability. No other instructors were telling me that food reactions could make people anxious and depressed or have other physical and mental symptoms. I set this episode aside in my mind and forgot about it until years later.

In 1952, I was a first-year resident in psychiatry. Walter Alvarez, M.D., had just written a book entitled *The Neuroses*. As a fledgling psychiatrist, naturally I was interested in learning from this honored, successful internist of the Mayo Clinic. To my surprise, he devoted several pages to describing headaches, dulling of the brain, and other emotional reactions as precipitated by allergies to certain foods. None of my psychiatry instructors had pointed out to me any cases with symptoms related to allergic reactions to foods or chemicals. In fact, I thought Dr. Alvarez wasn't very wise, that as an internist he didn't know enough about psychiatry, and that he had made an error in judgment. After all, wasn't it the hostility for father, mother, brother, sister, or uncle that caused the headache, depression, or mental confusion? I set his ideas aside because they did not seem true. Certainly nothing in my training was telling me otherwise. So again, I forgot the entire matter until years later.

In 1966, my friend Joseph Wolpe, M.D., sent me a copy of a paper by allergist Theron G. Randolph, M.D., which had been presented at a medical meeting in London. Dr. Wolpe knew that I was interested in tracing possible organic factors in mental illness and suggested that I might be interested in the paper. To my amazement, Dr. Randolph described the following as occurring during allergy food tests administered to patients: mania, depression, and, indeed, all the classic neurotic and schizophrenic symptoms that my patients manifested. My response toward the contents of the paper was "incredible, impossible!" None of my patients were reacting to foods and chemicals. Instead, it seemed clear to me at the time that their symptoms were, by and large, related to more immediate life circumstances, or sometimes due to deficiencies that I could demonstrate by laboratory examinations. My attitude was that some day, when I had plenty of time, I would restudy the paper, but during that period of my life it didn't seem all that important.

In 1970, at the advice of S. Klotz, M.D., I read a book entitled *Food Allergy* by Rinkel, Randolph, and Zeller. This book claimed that after four days of fasting, foods could be clinically assessed on an induction-test basis with symptoms disappearing during a period of four days' avoidance and reappearing when tested with meals of single foods. Headache, depression, feeling drugged, insomnia, tension, hallucinations, delusions, paranoia, catatonia, and other symptoms were described as having been observed during induction food testing.[6]

Herbert Rinkel, M.D., the senior author, had a personal experience that led him to examine more closely the possibilities of symptom formation due to foods. At the allergy clinic, some of the staff had prepared him a birthday cake. Within a few minutes of eating a piece of it, he fell to the floor, unconscious. When he came to, he asked what had happened. He was curious enough to assess the contents of the angel food cake and discovered that the only food it contained that he had not eaten during the past four days was egg. He usually ate at least one egg a day because his parents lived on a farm and supplied him with free eggs; however, he had run out of eggs four days before. He discovered that he was able to reproduce the unconscious state he had experienced by avoiding eggs for four days and then allowing himself a single exposure. This experience led him to examine the relationship of food symptoms revealed in all his patients.

I then studied *Allergy of the Nervous System* by Frederic Speer, M.D., an allergist at the University of Kansas.[7] The book pulls together evidence from allergy and neurological literature indicating that emotional and neurological symptoms have been observed and recorded since the 1920s. The book gives case histories of patients with the classic psychotic states that psychiatrists diagnose as schizophrenia. Through the years I encountered works by Drs. Rowe, Duke, Crowe, Kennedy, Davidson, Alvarez, Clark, Rinkel, Randolph, Mandell, and a number of others, describing emotional and neurological reactions as responses to selective exposure of foods and chemicals. How could I say, I asked myself, that all these doctors were wrong and that they just didn't know enough about psychiatry? After reading the overwhelming evidence, I developed the conviction that I, too, should take these reactions into account in my diagnoses, and let the evidence, rather than prejudice, speak for itself.

"We doctors," writes Dr. Alvarez, "are the most stubborn lot in the world! Many doctors are so stubborn as to think that a fact can't be true if they were not taught it in medical school."[8] I was taught to take a history of a psychiatric patient's life, examine his symptoms, especially in terms of content, and from this deduce their cause, based on the doctrine that the mind can influence the body and that unhealthy emotions can result from disturbed interpersonal relationships and stressful incidents in the patient's life. I was also taught that psychiatry encompasses the broad spectrum of behavioral needs. Historically, it is as strongly rooted in philosophy as it is in physical science. To a great extent, diagnoses are based on clusters of symptoms and not on their cause. The depressed, anxious, and phobic person is diagnosed as neurotic. The delusional, perceptually distorted, hallucinating, and confused person is diagnosed as psychotic and usually labeled with the term *schizophrenic.* Psychiatry's strong philosophical bias leads to the basic assumption that, with rare exceptions, these neurotic and psychotic symptoms stem from the emotions of a biologically intact person. It is clearly understood that a range of minor and major behavioral symptoms may have organic causes, but the underlying concept remains that the majority of behavioral problems do not arise from these organic causes but rather from an assortment of conflicts, hostilities, guilt, dependencies, personality immaturities, and so forth. This bias toward philosophical causes has created a situation in which the majority of behavioral problems are not seriously subjected to a differential diagnosis based on a full range of organic causes.

There are models of psychosis, such as symptoms induced by LSD or amphetamines; however, we know that in most cases our schizophrenic patients have not been taking LSD or amphetamines, and therefore we say this is only a model of psychosis—something like, but not the same as, the real thing. The question arises: If we know the substances to which a person is reacting maladaptively, is it possible to treat his specific disorder in the same way as we would LSD- or amphetamine-induced illness? Allergists are giving us evidence that this is true, and that the substances involved are the foods the patient frequently eats and the chemicals he commonly encounters. Thus we are learning from the allergist-ecologist that induction allergy tests on psychiatric patients are feasible and worthwhile; we must conclude that to induce a symptom and be able to turn it on and turn it off is more impressive than philosophical reasoning.

It became evident to me that medicine at large has been negligent in examining the ecologic-organic evidence of food and chemical allergies as causes in both physical and mental illness. In fact, ecologic allergy examination on a broad spectrum is not taught to doctors in any specialty and especially in psychiatry. I began to realize that there needs to be added to the patient's history, physical examination, and laboratory diagnosis a broad-spectrum ecologic diagnosis, that is, the patient as she is, defective or otherwise, reacting to her total environment. This is a basic building block of preventive medicine. If such an ecologic examination for food and chemical allergies were introduced into the basic practice of medicine, it would revolutionize diagnosis and treatment. According to Randolph—and my experience bears this out—more than half of the so-called psychosomatic reactions are in reality undiagnosed allergic reactions. Doctors do not know this because they have not been taught how to make such an examination; thus, the causes of these reactions have remained a mystery to them. Psychiatry offers them the psychosomatic explanation, and because it is true that the mind can influence the body, it is assumed that this is what is happening, without making a reasonable differential diagnosis, which could prove whether that is in fact the case. Now, however, a method is available by which we may watch the symptoms leave by avoidance and emerge on exposure. Therefore, we are in a position to engage less in guesswork and more in immediate clinical diagnosis and management of the specific allergic reactions.

In his foreword to Dr. Speer's *Allergy of the Nervous System*, Dr. Alvarez describes a personal experience which parallels Dr. Rinkel's allergic response to eggs.[9] As a young man, Dr. Alvarez made a trip lasting several days into the mountains and on his return was very hungry. He ate an entire boiled chicken. In a few hours, he developed severe diarrhea, his brain was so dulled he could not read with comfort, and he suffered visual hallucinations of a strange, new world of many colors. These symptoms lasted for four days, then disappeared. If Walter Alvarez had been taken to a psychiatrist in this acute state of mental disorder, what would the diagnosis have been? Schizophrenia, almost certainly—and no psychiatrist would have thought to relate this eating of chicken to the symptoms. Fortunately for him, he did not go to a psychiatrist. As a young internist he had pieced together the relationship between chicken allergy and his symptoms; he stopped eating chicken. He became one of America's efficient and honored diagnosticians; but if he had continued to eat chicken, even as much as twice a week, he might well have been sitting in the back ward of a state hospital, subject to visual hallucinations, unable to read, and afraid of the world. "Certain it is," he writes, "that the psychiatrist and the allergist should work together for the solution of their more difficult problems."[10]

I would like to submit to you that there are thousands of people like Dr. Alvarez who, if they would omit from their diet, or space in their diet on a rotation basis, foods to which they are symptom reactive, could be socially and professionally efficient, honored, and successful, but who, if they continue frequent contact with these foods, can become psychotic, with life passing them by. "A number of other allergists," writes Howard Rapaport, "have documented the many mental symptoms and behavioral problems that are caused by food additives and food allergies. If mental illness caused by allergies were recognized more, and emotional factors not always sought to explain mental disturbances, a great deal of time and money could be saved, and patients' mental conditions eliminated. There are millions of patients enduring needless suffering."[11]

I believe it is time to sort out such people by allergy induction testing and give them a chance. It is my conviction that diagnoses such as "schizophrenic," "manic-depressive," and other psychotic, neurotic, or psychosomatic labels are relatively meaningless and tend only to aggravate the illness. It is the underlying organic cause that is important. We should be diagnosing paranoia caused by a wheat allergy, dissociation as a manifestation of a sensitivity to eggs, catatonia as a manifestation of mold or hydrocarbon allergy, and so forth, according to people's specific reactions to individual foods, chemicals, and inhalants. We psychiatrists need to scrap our archaic method of philosophical-psychiatric diagnosis. In general medical practice today, we doctors examine cause-and-effect relationships, such as pneumonia being caused by a specific organism and treatable by a specific antibiotic to which the organism is susceptible. It is my observation and belief that psychiatric diagnosis and treatment can be subjected to the same kind of scientific study the rest of medicine utilizes in diagnosis and treatment. Induction allergy testing, rather than deductive reasoning, I believe, is the method that will allow psychiatrists to function not as philosophers but as true scientists.

Chapter 3

Human Ecology and Mental Health

Hans Selye taught us that chronic stress, physical or emotional, leads to chronic illness, physical or emotional. Of the many stresses that plague mankind, the linked ones of allergic and addiction reactions are of the greatest intensity and most prolonged, and therefore are frequently central causes of physical or emotional symptoms, either temporary or chronic.

The extent and nature of such stresses vary markedly from person to person. The individual's ability to handle toxins, pollens, foods, and chemicals contracted from the environment differs considerably according to his unique chemical makeup. The more defective his ability, by inheritance, enzyme deficiency, malnutrition, harbored infection, or otherwise, the more likely a person is to develop maladaptive symptoms on exposure to food and environmental contacts. Our peculiar cultural preferences for eating only a few types of foods, heavy consumption of refined carbohydrates, and the chronic use of alcohol and tobacco add materially to a developing state of nutritional deficiency with its corresponding multiple-symptom production in our body-tissue systems. Also, our nation's propensity to consume nutritionally deficient "junk foods" further increases the defective tissue states in the human body. These defective tissue states undermine an individual's ability to handle without symptom formation the contacts he has with toxins, pollens, foods, and chemical fumes. Whether we choose to call these reactions toxic, allergic, allergic-like, or maladaptive is immaterial. The significant facts are:

1. Reaction by symptom formation occurs between the relatively intact human organism and its environmental contacts.
2. These reactions are consistent and therefore reproducible by anyone who follows the known rules for evoking symptoms.
3. The greater the defectiveness of the organism, the greater the likelihood of such maladaptive reactions occurring.
4. Any system that favorably improves the state of tissue health or the general homeostatic state of the organism by specific means (better nutrition, avoidance of incriminated substances, enzyme therapy, or meganutrient therapy) reduces the occurrence of these undesirable reactions and is, therefore, valid as a methodology.

In a total context of symptom causes, how important are these maladaptive food and chemical reactions? Theron Randolph, M.D., initially trained in both internal medicine and allergy, considers that 60 to 70 percent of symptoms diagnosed as psychosomatic are in fact undiagnosed maladaptive reactions to foods, chemicals, and inhalants. My own practice as a psychiatrist has shown that for 250 consecutive, unselected emotionally disturbed patients, there is convincing evidence that the majority developed major symptoms on exposure to their commonly consumed foods and frequently encountered chemicals. The highest percentage of symptom formation occurred in those diagnosed as psychotic. Ninety-two percent of those classified as schizophrenic developed symptoms as maladaptive reactions to foods and chemicals; 64 percent manifested symptom formation on exposure to wheat; 51 percent manifested symptom formation on exposure to mature corn products; and 51 percent manifested symptom formation on exposure to pasteurized whole cow's milk. Approximately 75 percent of the schizophrenics manifested symptom formation to tobacco; 10 percent of this group became grossly psychotic, with a paranoid reaction being the most common type of symptom formation in tobacco psychosis. Approximately 30 percent developed symptoms on exposure to petrochemical hydrocarbons. Some of the reactions in this group were so severe as to precipitate suicidal attempts or delusions.

The emotional symptoms evoked on exposure to foods and commonly met chemicals range from mild central-nervous-system symptoms such as weakness, dizziness, blurred vision, anxiety and depression, paranoid delusions, and visual and auditory hallucination. I do not recall any schizophrenic symptom described in the medical literature that was not observed in the 250 patients tested; gross psychotic symptoms occurred in a very high percentage.

The group also displayed physical reactions to an even greater extent. Headaches, dizziness, unsteadiness, inability to read or write, neuritis, myalgia, arthralgia, tension, hyperactivity, weakness, sleepiness, insomnia, tachycardia, gastritis, diarrhea, colitis, constipation, hypertension, hypotension, itching, hives, psoriasis, seborrhea, and many other such reactions were observed.

Cereal-grain psychosis

Henry, seventeen years old, had been mentally ill for three years. Prior use of tranquilizers, psychotherapy, and electric shock did not succeed in helping him appreciably. He believed that people were out to kill him, and he often had to be placed under restraint because of his attacks on innocent children and adults. He was placed on a fast from all foods and given spring water only. He remained mentally ill until the fourth day, at which time his symptoms cleared; he was released from his restraints. He telephoned his parents, saying, "I love you. Please come and see me." On the fifth day of the fast he was fed a meal of wheat only. Within an hour, he began to feel strange and unreal; within an hour and a half, he thought people were going to kill him. He telephoned his parents again, saying, "I hate you. You caused my illness. I don't want to ever see you again." Further testing confirmed the fact that when specific foods were withheld, his symptoms cleared, and when given wheat again the same paranoid reaction occurred consistently.

This was one of the early cases of my clinical ecology studies of central-nervous-system reaction to foods. How could it be with all my years of psychiatric specialty training and experience that I had never heard of or seen a case of paranoid schizophrenia caused by a specific food? What was this strange, new cereal-grain psychosis? It was difficult to admit, but here was a case of paranoid schizophrenia produced "by bread alone." Moreover, the illness could clearly be reproduced and observed by anyone who followed the regimen of four days off wheat followed by a meal of wheat only. At this stage of my experience, all I could honestly do was admit it was so, and admit the validity of those allergist-ecologists who reported observing such reactions while test-exposing patients to foods. Later, I was encouraged by the fact that others were experiencing similar reactions in their patients. F. C. Dohan, for example, observed in a study published in 1973 that there were a substantially significant group of schizophrenics whose symptoms relate to reactions to cereal grains. Schizophrenics sufficiently ill to be locked in a ward, who had cereal grains and dairy products removed from their diets, were compared with a similar, equal-sized group allowed cereal grains and milk. Those with cereal grains and dairy products removed from their diets were released from the ward in half the time required for those not so treated. When gluten from wheat was secretly added to their diets, these patients became ill again.

Another Jesus Christ?

Karl had been under treatment for paranoid schizophrenia; tranquilizers had been used with only partial success. Periodically, he thought he was Jesus Christ and that his father was God. He was afraid someone would injure his small son; consequently, he would take the boy and run away from other people. During these episodes, he would suddenly fear that he would hurt his son and would quickly give the child to whoever was nearby.

The morning of his first day in the hospital he exhibited his usual symptoms; however, he also complained of smelling gas. Based on my psychiatric training, I reasoned that this was another of Karl's delusions. I had seen many schizophrenics who said they smelled various things; I always assumed their ideas to be delusions. But by now, my clinical-ecological experience had made me question the validity of my medical training. I began to look for a source of gas, for I knew that any person with a lowered biochemical homeostasis with a prior record of maladaptive allergic reactions to either foods or chemicals would be much more sensitive to the incriminating substance or substances than, for example, I would. Therefore, he or she would recognize the presence of the substance in the environment long before I would.

It turned out that across from his room was a dumbwaiter going to the kitchen below. Around the corner from his room was a stairway leading to the kitchen. I opened the door to the stairway, and to my surprise I, too, smelled gas. They had just cooked breakfast on a gas range below. He was right! He did smell gas; his hypersensitivity at detecting the presence of natural gas was acute because he was allergic to this substance.

I placed him in another room that was free from any gases or other pollutants. He was also put on a fast, drinking spring water only. Each day I asked him about his symptoms. On the morning of the fourth day his symptoms were gone. I took him to our allergy-test room and, without telling him the substance I was using, placed drops of auto-exhaust-fume extract under his tongue for quick absorption into his system. In about two minutes or so he announced to me that he was Jesus Christ. I gave him 100 percent oxygen to breathe for five minutes. When this did not help, I added a small amount of CO_2 to the oxygen; CO_2 improves the body's use of oxygen. After about two minutes of breathing oxygen and carbon dioxide, he announced that he was not Jesus Christ.

I had turned off his delusion by arranging for the avoidance of contact with petroleum products; then, when he was symptom-free, I exposed him to exhaust-fume extract, which induced the symptoms within minutes. I again turned off the delusion, this time through the detoxifying effect of oxygen and carbon dioxide. The fundamental cause of the psychotic delusion was no longer a mystery.

His history revealed that three years before, while driving a propane-fueled fork truck in an apple warehouse cooler, he was overcome by the fumes from the truck, fell to the floor, and was revived by emergency oxygen. It was after this that he developed his psychosis, and these attacks had always coincided with his driving the fork truck in the apple cooler. He also reacted to several foods, but only gas fumes made him delusional. It was significant that, on one occasion when he waxed his crew-cut hair, he literally went crazy. People who are very sensitive to petrochemical hydrocarbons have to avoid items coming from petroleum sources: candles, waxes, sprays, fresheners, perfumes, certified food coloring, exhaust fumes, whitened cane sugar, and anything else derived from or contaminated by petrochemical hydrocarbons.

Approximately one-third of my patients react to various chemicals common to our environment. Some react to the insecticide spray residues on fruits and vegetables and thus must eat fruits and vegetables that have not been sprayed by insecticides if they are to remain sane. Some react to preservatives and additives in foods; others react to the noncaking substance in table salt and have to use sea salt. Another surprise was the number of people reacting to chlorinated water; several developed ulcerated colitis. I had never heard of chlorine as a cause of either ulcerated colitis or psychosis, but my empirical observations made me a believer.

There were many other patients who manifested a variety of severe maladaptive reactions to foods and chemicals. A twenty-year-old paranoid schizophrenic became symptom-free by the fourth day of a fast on spring water only. When test smoking a cigarette, he became disoriented and delusional and defied anyone to come near him. It took four men to subdue him and place him in a seclusion room. He had been well until two years before when he began smoking. A fifty-two-year-old woman with a neurotic depression was tested for wheat. She developed a stiff neck and tightness in the chest and throat; even worse, she felt like hitting or punching someone. She was so frightened she might act on these compulsive urges that she went to a room by herself until the reaction subsided.

A twelve-year-old boy diagnosed as hyperkinetic had the following symptoms on testing for spinach: he became overtalkative and physically violent, had excessive saliva, was very hot, developed a severe stomachache, and cried for a long time. Watermelon made him irritable and depressed; cantaloupe made him aggressively tease other patients. Once he avoided the incriminating substances in his diet, his hyperkinesis symptoms diminished dramatically.

Pineapple evoked irritability, blocking of thought, dizziness, and a severe headache in a thirty-six-year-old psychoneurotic woman. Oranges made her violently angry, and she fought with her son; her mind functioned so poorly she could hardly carry on a conversation. Rice brought on uncontrollable giggling followed by crying.

A four-year-old boy diagnosed as hyperkinetic had a variety of reactions. String beans made him hyperactive, and he wanted to fight with everyone. Celery gave him a severe stomachache, after which he cried and became grouchy. Strawberries made him angry and hyperactive and caused a great deal of coughing. Unrefined cane sugar caused him to be irritable, after which he coughed and developed a stuffy nose.

A forty-year-old schizophrenic woman responded to a sublingual test for petrochemical hydrocarbons using glycerinated exhaust fumes by trying to find a way to kill herself. She had a history of attempting suicide by opening the door of the car and trying to jump out while her husband was driving. She would act normally when starting on a ride, but within a few minutes she would try to hurl herself from the car and have to be restrained by her husband.

He later discovered the car had a faulty exhaust system, which had been leaking fumes into its interior.

A twelve-year-old boy became listless and depressed, and cried when tested for bananas. Then he became aggressive and picked up a stick as if to hit another patient. When he ate oranges, he sang at first but then became very tired, impatient, and eventually wild and aggressive. Rice caused him to experience a sensation of heat, followed by rebellious hyperactivity.

I could go on and on with case histories that reveal the evidence that objectively observed induction testing of foods and chemicals reveals the cause-and-effect relationship between maladaptive reactions to foods and chemicals and psychotic aggressive behavior, as well as numerous other physical and central-nervous-system reactions. But let us for a minute move directly into the subjective, real world of a cerebral central-nervous-system-allergy patient. Here is a firsthand account of the horror experienced by one of my patients during a lifetime of misery and mental anguish. Mary writes:

> I guess it's the way it suddenly came over me that frightened me so much. To feel fine one minute and the next have the world crumbling around you is enough to scare anyone. What had I done to bring this on myself? An endocrinologist suggested I could control it, because it really must all be psychological. He suggested that I see a psychiatrist. Imagine: a seventy-dollar visit to a specialist who says, "It's really all in your head and you should see a psychiatrist."
>
> I had no way of knowing that this November was going to be any different from any other November except that I seemed much more tired than usual. Household chores became a sheer act of will. My supper alarm soon became the initial step that led me to walking into the walls, tripping over familiarly placed furniture, and a sick feeling in the pit of my stomach. What was going to become of me?
>
> Finally the horror would come. And so, insidiously, would a feeling of sweeping closeness. It was getting very warm. My dry lips were aware of my hot and cold clammy face and hands. My eyes would experience a flashing strobe-light sensation. Here, it

was coming, shallow at first, as if to gain one's composure. Then, it came more rapidly and a little more frantic. "I can't breathe . . . please, God, someone help me. I'm going to pass out. . . . My arms and legs are going weak with needles and pins. My heart is pounding and my rapid pulse is bulging over 120 beats per minute. Please, God . . . air, a window, a chair to sit down a while, a few minutes to reestablish reality!" It's finally over, and I am exhausted. Exhausted by an unknown experience that would wake me out of a sound sleep or catch me in a rush on my way to lunch. Where would I find the answer, the explanation for all this?

"Well, dearie, you were just meant to be a big girl," said the first six doctors. They were referring, of course, to my weight problem. When asked about my blood pressure dropping from 120/80 to 80/40 or my pulse soaring from 80 beats per minute to 120 to 140, their reply would be: "We really don't understand low blood pressure and the resultant rapid pulse."

Was it really true that God had intended me to be fat and miserable both? Was this really my bag of rocks to carry? Who could sympathize with such an unglamorous, boring plight? But then my November introduced me to Dr. William Philpott, the psychiatrist. Why not a psychiatrist? Everything had failed miserably.

Is this guy for real? I asked. What does he mean, he wants to know what food I am eating in my diet? How come he doesn't ask me about my perfectly happy marriage, and my two loving parents who struggled all their lives in order that "me and mine" might have a better time of it? How is it possible that he understands my dire exhaustion or my passing feeling of self-destruction, which at times seemed to be the only way to effect relief from my nightmare? How is it that this doctor's inventory question sheet resembles my diary: afraid and nervous about everything, on edge, impatient, and suffering from a totally jangled nervous system?

"A four-day fast," he says, "will find you feeling much better." It did, amazingly enough! "This morning," he asks, "how do you feel?" "Dr. Philpott, I feel the best I have felt in years." Dr. Philpott outlined my schedule: I was going to be tested for food allergy and hopefully it would show the effect, if any, a particular food had on my entire system rather than just my skin. In the meantime, my complete physical workup had been finished, and it showed very unhealthy low percentages that would require supplemental vitamins, minerals, amino acids, and enzymes.

A quart of milk, sipped in stages, immediately produced the horror of my aforementioned reactions. They were reproduced by evaporated milk, cheddar cheese, American cheese, cottage cheese, and so forth. My dairy product meals were interrupted by other testing meals of fruits and vegetables, none of which yielded the same reaction, except for chocolate, which produced a viselike temporal headache. The chocolate, I might add, was one of the testing foods administered to me via sublingual drops, which had no flavor. I can actually and honestly state here that I had eaten foods, totally unaware of their content. As before, I have no voluntary control over these reactions. However, I find that I can actually turn my symptoms on with and off without the use of milk, dairy products, or chocolate—truly amazing!

Ironically, it seems that each time I narrowed down my intake for weight-loss purposes (as the prior six doctors said I must), I unknowingly narrowed it down to include the things to which I am allergic. And, in my case, abstinence produces a reaction-free state. I feel great! This time I will not fail.

I think it's interesting to note that after following orthomolecular-ecological treatment, I was also able to become pregnant. Also interesting is the fact that my nursing baby breaks out in patches of eczema whenever I indulge, unwisely of course, in ice cream or chocolate. My withdrawal renders her skin clear in a matter of hours. However, my persistence finds itchy patches thriving. Interesting, when you stop and think about it—isn't it?[12]

The experience this case history describes is not uncommon. Mary is now a vivacious, outgoing, trusting, energetic, clearheaded person. It was easy for her to reduce and maintain an optimum weight after isolating the food allergies. She was sterile while reacting to foods and fertile when the foods were avoided and appropriate supplements (according to her laboratory-demonstrated needs) added. She does not have to be emotionally ill, depressed, sterile, fat, and wishing for death. The foods she eats and the frequency with which she eats them make the difference. Mary now knows how to live and stay symptom-free because she understands the cause-and-effect relationships between her environment and herself. Like many others on the same orthomolecular-ecologic metabolic program, there is little chance that she will ever need to return to the hospital. However, others with the same symptoms and diagnosis treated with electric shock, tranquilizers, antidepressants, and psychotherapy characteristically have repeated hospitalizations. Comparison studies of patients treated in these two different ways reveals this difference.

The anatomy of allergy-addiction

The chronic physical and mental reactions described in these case histories were observed to fade in intensity, and often to disappear completely, on a four-day fast and complete avoidance of chemicals, then to reemerge acutely on exposure to test meals of foods or chemicals of different kinds. They provide impressive evidence of having actually, under controlled experimental conditions, turned off an illness, while knowing why, and having turned the illness on again—and knowing why. But the question remains: What relationship does a period of four days have to an allergic reaction? Why should the avoidance of a chemical or certain food for a specific period result in a severe allergic symptom when a sensitive person is exposed to that chemical or food after the period of avoidance? The answers to these questions lie in a proper understanding of addiction and maladaptive allergic reactions.

Addiction is described as a state involving withdrawal-phase symptoms of any kind occurring hours or days (up to three days) after contact with a particular substance. Similarly, these withdrawal-phase symptoms can often be stopped—sometimes only partially—by continued contact with the addictive substance. Foods of all kinds, as well as chemicals, qualify as much as addictants as do narcotics, tobacco, coffee, and alcohol. But for our purposes of explanation, tobacco allergy-addiction can be cited as a model. Since about 75 percent of all people are allergic to tobacco, their first contact occasions immediate allergic symptoms: usually nausea, dizziness, and/or a cough. With frequent use, these symptoms are suppressed by the tobacco contact and later emerge, if there is not continued use of tobacco, as withdrawal symptoms. These symptoms can be suppressed only if the tobacco is contacted frequently enough to keep the user in a relief or postponed state. This state of partial and temporary relief by contact with the allergen is termed "addiction." Understanding addiction as an extension of a maladaptive allergic-like state is necessary if one is to understand the seriousness of the addiction to frequently eaten foods and commonly met chemicals that plagues about 80 percent of mankind.

Adaptive addiction can be described as a state of relative freedom from symptoms, occasioned when the addictive substance is contacted frequently enough and the biological homeostatic state is in good repair. It is, however, a state of chronic stress, precariously balanced, and paves the way for the emergence of an "illness"—an acute allergic reaction previously described—upon the addition of stress of any kind. Such last-straw stresses may be:

- an overload of the allergen
- the addition of seasonal allergens such as pollens or other environmental stresses
- physical stresses such as excessive cold, heat, or fatigue
- harbored infections
- emotional stress

The person suffering from adaptive addiction may be likened to one walking a tightrope, from which he may easily fall at any time. If the patient falls from the tightrope—that is, develops an illness—solving that immediate stress, physiological or psychological, merely restores him to the adaptive-addictive tightrope, leaving him prey of any wind of stress that blows in his life. However, if the basic addiction is handled, he then has a broad base from which to handle all stress—he is on firm ground, so to speak, and off the tightrope. It is in this sort of situation that psychiatrists so frequently give only a partial answer to their patients' needs—tranquilizers, antidepressants, and so on—solving a little conflict here and there but failing to solve the basic underlying metabolic problem of allergy-addiction to foods and chemicals.

Dr. Randolph has clinically demonstrated that when there is a break in exposure to addictive substances of any kind for at least four days (it seems to take at least four days for any food or chemical to be entirely eliminated from the human system), then the addictive-adaptive reaction is converted to an immediate reaction with an allergic-like quality upon renewed exposure to the substance. This is in fact not a new discovery: Hippocrates reports in his writings the knowledge that if a food was avoided for as much as four days, a reexposure to that food might create a severe reaction in certain people. And this point cannot be overemphasized: All addictions display this pattern, whether they are narcotic, alcohol, tobacco, food, or chemical in source. In our clinic, we have observed that removing the patient for four or more days from contact with any suspected food or chemical addictive substances, and then selectively reexposing him to one substance at a time has produced the emergence of every shade of symptom described as schizophrenic, neurotic, or character neurotic, plus a host of common somatic symptoms often classed as psychosomatic. Such allergic-like reactions can either excite or inhibit any tissues or organs in the body and are, therefore, capable of giving rise to any set of symptoms these tissues are able to produce. This type of maladaptive reaction has been called "the great masquerader"; depression, hallucinations, delusions, perceptual distortions, catatonia, flatness of affect, hyperkinesis, and so forth, are all such frequently encountered maladaptive reactions as to justify the conclusion that the search for an allergic-addictive source must be considered a valid procedure in all differential diagnoses of such symptoms.

Further considerations of the four-day period of avoidance

During the first two or three days of a fast, symptoms often emerge. This is not caused by a starving need for nutrients, but by the withdrawal-phase symptoms of an addiction. A person without food addictions will not display symptoms on a four-day period of avoidance.

Usually by the fourth day of the fast such symptoms will have materially subsided or disappeared. If they have not subsided by the fourth day, the period of avoidance should be extended by one to three days to see if the patient improves. In some of the more severely allergic cases, four days on a fast is not enough for the symptoms to clear, and the fast can be extended up to seven days. This type of program is indicated for some chronically depressed or severely paranoid patients. It should be remembered that if there is not adequate environmental control, symptoms may continue because of exposure to a substance (e.g., smoke, gas, hydrocarbon pollution) to which the person is reacting.

Asthmatics, epileptics, diabetics on insulin, and markedly debilitated patients should be tested and treated under direct medical supervision. On the withdrawal of food, as well as the reentry of foods as test meals, asthmatic attacks or seizures can be evoked in susceptible people. Emotional reactions in food-sensitive persons during the fast and also during the food testing can range from mild—such as tension, fatigue, headache, dizziness—to marked psychotic states involving deep depression and a wish to die, hallucinations, delusions, and illogical aggression. Therefore, it is advised that when fasting and testing an emotionally disturbed person, an objective observer be available so that emergency medical help can be obtained if needed. It helps to realize that the symptoms occurring during the food testing are likely to subside in one to three hours, although in some cases it may be as much as five hours, and occasionally reactions have lasted up to three days. In these more severe cases, medical assistance to stop the reaction is indicated. The method by which this is accomplished will be discussed later. However, in most cases the symptoms will fade in a short time.

Water that is not chemically treated (i.e., spring, well, distilled, or filtered water) is used during testing since some people are known to react to chlorine and/or fluorine. There must be no smoking during the period of avoidance or the subsequent test days. If symptom-free by the fourth day of the fast, tobacco can be tested if desired. This is achieved by chain-smoking as quickly as possible a maximum of six cigarettes. The test ends as soon as symptoms develop. Dizziness, nausea, and weakness are common minor symptoms of tobacco allergy, but in a few patients (about 10 percent of schizophrenics) frank psychosis develops. If the person will agree to stop smoking without such a test, this is the better plan. Some people will remember the symptoms that developed when they smoked their first cigarette. When they are informed that this is evidence of allergy to tobacco, that is sufficiently convincing for these people to stop smoking. These are the lucky ones, for there is always the danger during the tobacco test of judgment being affected or aggressive behavior flaring up. But if the patient has to be convinced that he is tobacco-allergic, then the test must be done.

In any food-allergy-testing program, a comprehensive environmental control plan is vital. The purpose of environmental control is to isolate the person from all substances to which he may be reacting: fumes, animal dander, cosmetics, hair conditioners, perfumes, gas, air pollution containing industrial waste, dye odors, certain soaps used for cleaning, oil or gas from furnaces, moth balls, spray fresheners, and so forth. Obviously, it is much easier to arrange for an adequate environmental control in a hospital setting where a unit has been especially designed for this purpose; in some cases, this is an absolute necessity. If, during the fourth or fifth day of the fast, the pulse still remains high or there still remain ongoing common symptoms, then it is probably due to a lack of proper environmental control. In this case, the environment must be reexamined to see if there is some agent to which the person is reacting. The pulse should be below 85 before testing. The same withdrawal phase symptoms that occur with food addiction can occur on the second to third day of avoidance of incriminating environmental factors. This fact is important to remember, since in some cases the environmental factor is more of the culprit in the patient's illness than is his food.

If a person maladaptively reacts to a food when occasionally eaten, he is aware of this and hence does not like the food. Such reactions to infrequently eaten foods are rare and obviously are not associated with the chronic addictive state. A food has to be eaten two or more times a week to be addicting. The more frequently a food is eaten, the more likely it is to be incriminated in addiction. However, even though a food is infrequently eaten, it may belong to a family of which a member is frequently eaten, such as legumes, squash-melon-cucumber, dairy products, and gluten-bearing cereal grains (wheat, rye, oats, barley, corn). One member of a food family eaten frequently predisposes a person to maladaptive reactions to other members of the same family, even if infrequently eaten.

A choice has to be made as to the types of food to be tested:

- foods grown without insecticides
- market-grown foods which will contain insecticide residues
- raw foods
- cooked foods
- foods with preservatives and colors added

Theoretically, each of these categories needs to be tested separately. Sometimes a food can be eaten raw when it cannot be eaten cooked, or vice versa. Sometimes foods without spray residues can be eaten without a reaction. Sometimes there are reactions to food colors and food preservatives. The most practical way is to start with the foods as usually eaten which are market-grown fruits, vegetables, and meats, and the food eaten in the usual form, either cooked or raw. Definitive testing can then be done on those foods in which reactions occur. Colors and preservatives are left out of the initial food testing. If more than fifteen foods are reacted to, then insecticide residues should be suspected and several of the reactive foods retested from sources not containing insecticides. Ideal, but hard to achieve, is the initial testing of basic foods not containing insecticide residues, which, for certain patients, is a necessity.

Chapter 4

The Diversified Rotation Diet

After one has successfully diagnosed food or chemical maladaptive allergic reactions, the next obvious goal is to establish some kind of control whereby these reactions—and their associated addictions—can be completely avoided. The most reliable method of attaining this goal is a diversified rotation diet.

Though working out the details of this sort of diet takes considerable planning, the basic idea is simple: to remove certain foods and groups of foods—which are called "food families"—from the diet for a specified period in order to observe what reactions are produced by their withdrawal and reintroduction.

Allergist Fanny Lou Leeney, M.D., was the first to use this dietary approach. Allergist H. J. Rinkel, M.D., while practicing in Oklahoma City, Oklahoma, adopted the diversified rotation diet from Dr. Leeney. Using his understanding of masked food allergy or "food addiction," Dr. Rinkel demonstrated that a symptom-producing food does not have to be abandoned forever but can be returned to the diet after the body has had time to recover completely from the initial allergic reaction. Specifically, in order to stop the vicious cycle of addiction, foods that give minor reactions should be avoided for a minimum of three months; then they, too, should be eaten only once in four days. If reactions occur on this program, incriminated foods should be avoided for another two to three months and tried again. The principle here is to avoid the symptom-evoking substance until the refractory phase (i.e., that stage in which the allergic or allergic-like state is broken) of the healing process develops after a few days, weeks, or months. It is important that one realize that the refractory phase usually begins at about three weeks and is well established by three months of complete avoidance. No food addictions are likely to develop once the refractory stage has occurred and a four-day rotation diet is practiced.

In 1971, under the supervision of allergist Marshall Mandell, M.D., I started to test systematically patients by deliberate exposure to single foods. We found that a food fast using only nonchemically treated water gave us our best results of improvement as well as evidence of a cause-and-effect relationship between food addiction and symptom reactions. At this time, Randolph Theron, M.D., and Dr. Mandell advised a diversified rotation diet. Initially, this diet seemed so difficult that, for a number of patients, I used a method of allowing free and frequent use of their nonreactive foods (i.e., foods that produced no symptoms). A few months later, I readmitted several of these patients to the hospital. Retesting revealed they were again sick due to the establishment of new addictions to a new set of what were once nonreactive foods, which they now were eating frequently. It proved to be disastrous to allow frequent use of any foods. I therefore sought the most rigid separation of foods to prevent this reinstatement of addiction. In discussing my problem with several experienced ecologists, I adopted the advice of allergist John McLennon, M.D., who suggested that I keep the foods in families and space their contact four days apart. I asked Ruth Nielson, R.D., dietitian at Fuller Memorial Hospital where I was doing this work, to arrange diets with foods in families and with one food member per family to be eaten every four days.[13]

Foods, theoretically, should be rotated by families every four days, since there may be a cross-allergic reaction between family members. For example, lemon, orange, grapefruit, lime, tangerine, kumquat, and citron are all of the citrus family. If symptoms are evoked by this family of foods, then each food within the family should be first avoided for three months and then rotated on a four-day basis. That is, if I eat an orange on Monday, I should not eat any other member of the family until Friday of that same week. It is important to understand that even though this procedure requires specific dietary planning, which is often difficult to carry out, it does reduce allergic reactions as well as increase one's exposure to a broader spectrum of nutrients.

As the years progressed, I became convinced that the eating of only one member of a food family every four days was a very demanding regime and was not necessary for all my patients. As a result, I adopted a "maximum restrictive diversified rotation diet"—either on a four- or seven-day basis for the more severely allergic patient—and a "minimum restrictive four-day diversified rotation diet" for those who manifest less severe allergic or addictive responses.

Dr. Randolph has had the most years of experience in the area of diet and human ecology of any physician and therefore has been most meticulous in his application and observations of the diversified rotation diet. His maximum restrictive diversified rotation diet has become the standard of excellence in the field. His conclusions are that the most efficient program has three main points:

1. Any one food, whether initially symptom-reactive or not, should be eaten only once in four days.
2. Foods are established in families, with only one member of any family eaten during any one day.
3. One day must intervene between the use of any two members of a family.

For example, while wheat would not be eaten more frequently than once in four days, another member of this cereal-grain family, such as oats, could be eaten as a single meal on the third day of the rotation, with wheat again being eaten on the first day of the next cycle, the fifth day of the program. He also believes that the smaller the number of foods eaten in a single meal, the fewer the chances of a reaction occurring. Several foods may be eaten successfully by most people, but only one, two, or three foods at a meal may be necessary for a few severely sensitive reactors. This is probably caused by a selective inability of such a person to provide adequate digestive enzymes and/or other metabolic factors to handle the metabolism of the multiple foods.

Patients should be taught to return to the foods to which they were initially demonstrated to be symptom-reactive. It is important that they not try to do without these foods completely for the rest of their lives; often these are foods that are nutritionally valuable. If a patient finds that he cannot reinstate such a food after three months, he should try at four or five months. If he finds that he cannot rotate them once in four days, he should try once every eight days or once every two weeks or once a month.

A minority of subjects have, and a minority of foods cause, fixed food allergies. These are usually easy to spot because each time the person eats the food, symptoms develop in spite of avoidance and/or rotation. Certain incriminating chemicals fall into this category. In the case of fixed food or chemical allergy, the substance must be avoided completely at all times. Any type of program such as described above will not help a fixed food allergy; only complete avoidance will stop reactions in these cases.

There is no way other than rotation to assure a nonreactive state toward initially symptom-incriminated foods. However, there is some degree of protection provided by adequate nutrition. In examining patients, it is often demonstrated in the laboratory that they are deficient in vitamins C and B_6, folic acid, chromium, zinc, magnesium, manganese, and so forth. Providing these necessary nutrients, as well as others, is an aid in reducing the maladaptive reactivity to the foods. A detailed examination of these different orthomolecular aspects of treatment will be given in subsequent chapters, but for now let us always remember that the rotation diet is the first and most important weapon used in the battle against addictions.

Overview of the maximum restrictive diversified four-day rotation diet

1. Eat no single food more often than once in four days. This applies whether or not these foods were initially symptom-evoking.
2. Foods are classified by families so that members of a specific family will be used only on the days assigned to that family. (See "Maximum Restrictive Diversified Four-Day Rotation Diet" chart, page 42.)
3. There must be at least a one-day interval between uses of members of the same family.
4. The smaller the number of foods used in a single meal, the less chance of a maladaptive reaction. Some highly reactive people can eat only one, two, or three foods at a meal while less reactive people can eat a much greater variety at one time.
5. A large amount of food eaten increases the chance of a reaction. Therefore, moderate servings are preferable to large servings.

Other considerations

1. For some, allergic reactions will occur if a food is eaten on a single-exposure four-day rotation basis, whereas a reaction may not occur if spaced on a single-exposure eight-, sixteen-, or thirty-two-day basis.
2. Any time a food is suspected of evoking a symptom, it should be tested as a single meal on the next four-day cycle. If symptoms are evoked, it should be omitted for a minimum of six weeks and a maximum of twelve weeks and reintroduced into the rotation diet on a trial basis.

3. Some foods combined into a single meal may evoke symptoms when they do not do so as a single food or in combination with other foods. These types of reactions are best determined on an individual-tolerance basis.
4. Occasionally, highly sensitive persons have improved tolerance if exposures to specific foods are kept on a four-to-seven-day rotation combination. Thus, the sensitive reactor to wheat, corn, milk, and cheese may do well on a basic four-day rotation diet for all other foods, but must eat wheat, corn, milk, and cheese at a Saturday or Sunday meal only.
5. When reactions to a large assortment of foods occur, or when the evoking of symptoms is erratic, then the cumulative effect of insecticide residues should be suspected. This can be ruled in or out by test meals of several non-chemically contaminated foods and sublingual provocative tests on an assortment of insecticide sprays used on fruits and vegetables.
6. Some foods within the same family are sufficiently alike from a chemical standpoint that symptoms may occur even when rotated on a two-day basis. Examples are wheat, rye, oats, and similar gluten-containing foods. Buckwheat contains gluten even though it is not a member of the cereal-grain family. However, rice and millet, both of the cereal-grain family, do not contain gluten. Therefore, it is best to keep the gluten-containing cereal grains on a once-in-four-days basis and keep the non-gluten cereals on a two-day basis, such as rice two days after millet. My experience with this system gave satisfactory results.

I have not provided suggested menus for the following rotation diets, although I have prepared a number of them for my patients. The problem here is that a menu, once given, is all too likely to be followed rigorously, without regard to the individual's needs and tastes. Anyone wishing to use the following diets should understand:

1. Not all the food families given for each day need be employed on that day. For Day 1 of the first diet, there are twenty-eight food families listed; the idea of dutifully eating one member of each family is overwhelming. The idea is to restrict one's consumption for that day to the families listed, and to repeat no family more often than specified.
2. Any day's menus should have a reasonable balance of protein, fat, and carbohydrate, and should be as palatable and satisfactory as the given guidelines allow.

Overview of the minimum restrictive diversified four-day rotation diet

1. Foods are kept in families on a four-day basis. No member of the family is eaten more frequently than every four days.
2. Multiple foods from the same family can be used on the same day multiple times.
3. Foods not reacted to can be used multiple times on the same day.
4. If a food has been reacted to, use it only once in four days after the initial six- or twelve-week avoidance period.

This diet is the same as the maximum restrictive diversified four-day rotation diet, except that it permits multiple meals of members of the same family on that day prescribed for the specific family, providing that no initial reactions to these foods are present on provocative food testing, intradermal serial-dilution provocative testing, or cytotoxic or RAST testing.

Maximum Restrictive Diversified Four-Day Rotation Diet

	Food families	
Day 1	Rose	Strawberry, blackberry, loganberry, rose hip
	Grape	Grape, raisin
	Banana	Banana, plantain
	Apple	Apple
	Mulberry	Mulberry, breadfruit
	Potato	Potato, tomato, eggplant, peppers (red and green), chili pepper, paprika, cayenne, ground cherries
	Lily	Onion, chive, asparagus
	Fungus	Mushroom, yeast (brewer's yeast, baker's yeast, and such)
	Beet	Spinach
	Mallow	Okra, cottonseed
	Grass	Wheat, oats, rye, barley
	Buckwheat	Buckwheat, rhubarb
	Bovidae	Beef, milk, cheese, yogurt, butter
	Mollusca	Scallop, abalone, snail, squid, clam, mussel, oyster
	Salt-water fish	Mackerel, flounder, anchovy
	Walnut	Pecan
	Protea	Macadamia nut
	Leguma	Peanut
	Flaxseed	Flaxseed
	Laurel	Bay leaf, cinnamon
	Nutmeg	Nutmeg
	Arrowroot	Arrowroot
	Orchid	Vanilla
	Sterculia	Cocoa, chocolate
	Oil	Peanut, cottonseed
	Sweetener	Beet sugar, maple sugar
	Tea	Rose hip, strawberry leaf

Day 2	Bird	Chicken, quail, pheasant, and their eggs
	Plum	Plum, cherry, peach, almond
	Gourd	Watermelon, pumpkin, cucumber, acorn squash, pumpkin seed
	Citrus	Orange, lime
	Palm	Coconut, date
	Papaw	Papaw, papaya, papain
	Parsley	Carrot, parsnip, parsley, anise, dill, fennel, cumin, coriander, caraway
	Mustard	Watercress, brussels sprouts, collards
	Composites	Endive, escarole, artichoke, romaine, safflower, tarragon
	Rabbit	Rabbit
	Crustacea	Crab, crayfish, lobster
	Fresh-water fish	Sturgeon, herring, whitefish
	Cashew	Cashew
	Mint	Basil, sage, horehound, catnip, spearmint
	Myrtle	Clove, allspice
	Olive	Olives (black and green)
	Oil	Coconut, almond, olive
	Sweetener	Date sugar, fructose
	Tea	Spearmint, papaya
Day 3	Apple	Pear, quince
	Rose	Raspberry, boysenberry
	Heath	Blueberry, huckleberry, cranberry, wintergreen
	Gooseberry	Currant, gooseberry
	Ebony	Persimmon
	Mulberry	Fig
	Grass	Corn, rice, millet, cane sorghum
	Laurel	Avocado, sassafras
	Legume	Pea, black-eyed pea, green bean, soybean, lentil, field pea, kidney bean, lima bean, navy bean, pinto bean, wax bean, carob, alfalfa
	Goosefoot	Beet, chard, lamb's-quarters
	Bovida	Lamb
	Suidae	Pork

	Salt-water fish	Sea herring, cod, sea bass, sea trout, tuna, swordfish, sole
	Spurge	Tapioca
	Birch	Filbert, hazelnut
	Walnut	English walnut, hickory nut, black walnut
	Pepper	Black and white pepper
	Lily	Garlic, leek
	Oil	Soybean, avocado, corn
	Sweetener	Carob, dextrose, glucose, cane, molasses, sorghum
	Tea	Alfalfa, sassafras, raspberry leaf
Day 4	Citrus	Lemon, grapefruit, tangerine, kumquat, citron
	Gourd	Cantaloupe, honeydew, yellow squash, zucchini, squash seed
	Plum	Apricot, nectarine, wild cherry
	Cashew	Mango, pistachio
	Pineapple	Pineapple
	Honeysuckle	Elderberry
	Morning glory	Sweet potato
	Mustard	Turnip, radish, horseradish, chinese cabbage, broccoli, cauliflower, kale, kohlrabi, rutabaga, mustard
	Composites	Lettuce, chicory, dandelion, sunflower seed
	Parsley	Celery, celery seeds
	Mammal	Turkey, duck, goose, guinea
	Crustacea	Prawn, shrimp
	Fresh-water fish	Salmon, bass, perch
	Beech	Chestnut
	Pedalium	Sesame
	Brazil nut	Brazil nut
	Mint	Oregano, savory, peppermint, thyme, marjoram
	Nutmeg	Mace
	Oil	Sesame, sunflower
	Sweetener	Honey
	Tea	Peppermint, lemon balm

Limitations to consider when using the minimum restrictive diversified four-day rotation diet

1. Maladaptive reactions may develop to foods eaten at multiple meals during the same day. This is due to the cumulative effect of the second or third exposure on the same day. If this occurs, the food must be left out for six weeks, and when reintroduced into the diet, it should be used once in four days thereafter. Experience with this program reveals that only occasionally do maladaptive reactions develop. Remember, however, the more often specific foods are used, the more likely maladaptive reactions are to occur.
2. Rather than using the same food several times on the same day, it is a safer practice to use another member of the same family once on this same day. Thus, wheat, rye, or oats could be eaten on the same day but at separate meals. Some prefer a multiple-grain breakfast cereal or bread. If this is used, it is preferably used only once, and any member of the cereal-grain family it contains should be used neither during the rest of this day nor until the next four-day rotation cycle.

Alternative split-day minimum restrictive diversified four-day rotation diet

This method starts the rotation day with the evening meal. It allows for initially demonstrated nonreactive foods that have been eaten in the evening meal to be eaten also for breakfast the next morning and at noon. Such a diet is for the convenience of the patient and is often appreciated. For most patients who have tried it, there have been good results. It has the inherent danger, however, of multiple exposures of the same food in a twenty-four-hour period, which may cumulatively result in an acute reaction.

Minimum Restrictive Diversified Four-Day Rotation Diet

	Food families	
Day 1	Mulberry	Mulberry, fig, breadfruit
	Rose	Strawberry, raspberry, blackberry, dewberry, loganberry, youngberry, boysenberry, rose hip
	Grape	All varieties of grape and raisin, cream of tartar
	Potato	Potato, tomato, eggplant, peppers (red and green), pimento, chili pepper, paprika, cayenne, ground cherries
	Goosefoot	Beet, spinach, swiss chard, lamb's-quarters
	Composites	Lettuce, chicory, endive, escarole, artichoke, dandelion, tarragon, safflower
	Bovidae	Lamb, beef, milk products (butter, cheese, yogurt), goat, deer
	Mollusca	Abalone, snail, squid, clam, mussel, oyster, scallop
	Spurge	Tapioca
	Cashew	Cashew, pistachio, mango
	Protea	Macadamia nut
	Nutmeg	Nutmeg, mace
	Oil	Safflower
	Sweetener	Beet sugar, maple sugar
	Tea	Comfrey, strawberry leaf, raspberry leaf, rose hip
Day 2	Plum	Plum, cherry, peach, apricot, nectarine, almond, wild cherry
	Pineapple	Pineapple
	Papaw	Papaw, papaya, papain
	Myrtle	Guava, clover, allspice, clove, pimento
	Grass	Wheat, corn, rice, oats, barley, rye, wild rice, cane, millet, sorghum, bamboo shoot
	Parsley	Carrot, parsnip, celery, celery seed, celeriac, anise, dill, fennel, cumin, parsley, coriander, caraway
	Fungus	Mushroom, yeast (brewer's yeast, baker's yeast, and such)
	Mallow	Okra, cottonseed
	Bird	All fowl and game birds*: chicken, turkey, duck, goose, guinea, pigeon, quail, pheasant, and their eggs

**Duck, chicken, and turkey are in separate families but closely related; they may be eaten every second or third day.*

	Salt-water fish	Sea herring, anchovy, cod, sea bass, sea trout, mackerel, tuna, swordfish, flounder, sole
	Beech	Chestnut
	Brazil nut	Brazil nut
	Flaxseed	Flaxseed
	Pedalium	Sesame
	Orchid	Vanilla
	Sterculia	Cocoa, chocolate
	Sweetener	Cane sugar (raw), clover honey (if not used on Day 4)
	Tea	Papaya tea
Day 3	Apple	Apple, pear, quince
	Banana	Banana, plantain
	Arrowroot	Arrowroot
	Heath	Blueberry, huckleberry, cranberry, wintergreen
	Gooseberry	Currant, gooseberry
	Ebony	Persimmon
	Legume	Pea, black-eyed pea, dry bean, green bean, carob, soybean, lentil, licorice, peanut, alfalfa
	Laurel	Avocado, cinnamon, bay leaf, sassafras, cassia bud or bark
	Buckwheat	Buckwheat, rhubarb
	Lily	Onion, garlic, asparagus, chive, leek
	Crustacea	Crab, crayfish, lobster, prawn, shrimp
	Suidae	Pork
	Birch	Filbert, hazelnut
	Conifer	Pine nut
	Pepper	Black and white pepper, peppercorn
	Oil	Soybean, peanut, avocado
	Sweetener	Fructose, carob syrup
	Tea	Alfalfa, sassafras
Day 4	Gourd	Watermelon, cantaloupe, other melons
	Citrus	Lemon, orange, grapefruit, lime, tangerine, kumquat, citron
	Honeysuckle	Elderberry
	Palm	Coconut, date, date sugar

Morning glory	Sweet potato
Gourd	Cucumber, pumpkin, squash, zucchini, acorn, pumpkin or squash seeds
Mustard	Mustard, turnip, radish, horseradish, watercress, cabbage, kraut, chinese cabbage, broccoli, cauliflower, brussels sprouts, collard, kale, kohlrabi, rutabaga
Olive	Black or green olives
Fresh-water fish	Sturgeon, herring, salmon, whitefish, bass, perch
Walnut	English walnut, black walnut, pecan, hickory nut, butternut
Mint	Basil, sage, oregano, savory, horehound, catnip, spearmint, peppermint, thyme, marjoram, lemon balm
Tea	Kaffer
Oil	Coconut, olive oil, pecan
Sweetener	Date sugar, honey

Maximum restrictive seven-day diversified rotation diet

This rotation diet is to be used by those who have many severe allergies. Less frequent contacts with food should help their systems to clear faster. Only one contact with each food is allowed every seven days, and one must continue to rotate all foods in family groups. Any of the foods listed for a day may be used, but only one contact is permitted with each food. This is best accomplished by using two to five foods at one meal and not repeating these foods at the following meal.

There are some rare individuals who can eat only one food with each meal, since combinations of any type give rise to symptoms. In such cases, six meals may be consumed per day, keeping these individuals on a strict seven-day rotation program.

Heating food in oils reduces the absorption rate and hence reduces symptoms. Oils should be rotated; use corn, safflower, peanut, olive, soy, and cottonseed oils. Butter, lard, and other animal fats may also be used. Heating in a Chinese wok is ideal. For those very sensitive persons requiring foods heated in oils, a seven-day rotation diet is preferred. Frequent or continual use of foods heated in oil is not recommended, however, since this procedure can raise the patient's free fatty acids and triglycerides. At the present time, there is considerable debate in medical circles about the values of various percentages of dietary fat, protein, and carbohydrate. Nathan Pritikin, M.D., author of a best-selling work on diet, concludes from the medical literature that 10 percent fat, 10 percent protein, and 80 percent complex carbohydrate as total calories provides the optimum ratio for reversal of and protection from arteriosclerosis, when this regime is coupled with systematic exercise.[14] While this ratio can be taken as a valuable general guideline, it should be understood that these percentages were arrived at without benefit of laboratory demonstrations for individual nutritional needs and without taking into account the effects of nutritional supplementation.

It appears likely, for instance, that supplemental vitamin C and pyridoxine would serve as additional protection against the inflammation leading to atheromatous plaque formation, often associated with arteriosclerosis, no matter what the intake percentages of carbohydrates, proteins, or fats. It is also probable that for some individuals, preferred percentages of fat might be in the range of 10 to 15 percent, of protein 10 to 20 percent, and complex carbohydrates 60 to 80 percent. Extensive research needs yet to be done in this area.

Maximum Restrictive Seven-Day Diversified Rotation Diet

	Food families	
Day 1	Apple	Apple, pear, quince
	Mulberry	Mulberry, fig, breadfruit
	Honeysuckle	Elderberry
	Olive	Olives (black and green)

	Gooseberry	Currant, gooseberry
	Potato	Potato, tomato, eggplant, peppers (red and green), chili pepper, paprika, cayenne
	Lily	Onion, garlic, asparagus, chive, leek
	Grass	Wheat, corn, rice, oats, barley, rye, wild rice, cane, millet, sorghum, bamboo shoot
	Buckwheat	Buckwheat, rhubarb
	Bovidae	Milk products (butter, cheese, yogurt), beef and pure beef products, lamb
	Mint	Basil, savory, sage, oregano, horehound, catnip, spearmint, peppermint, thyme, marjoram, lemon balm
	Oil	Olive, corn, 100 percent corn oil margarine, butter
	Tea	Rose hip, strawberry leaf
	Juice	Juice may be made and used, without added sweeteners, from the following: fruits—any listed above in any combination desired; vegetables
Day 2	Citrus	Lemon, orange, kumquat, citron, grapefruit, lime, tangerine
	Parsley	Carrot, celeriac, parsley, anise, parsnip, celery, celery seed, dill, cumin, coriander, caraway, fennel
	Pepper	White pepper
	Nutmeg	Mace
	Walnut	English walnut, black walnut, pecan, hickory nut, butternut
	Bird	Chicken, goose, quail, and their eggs
	Oil	Fat from any bird listed above; oil from any nut listed above
	Sweetener	Orange honey (use sparingly)
	Tea	Comfrey, comfrey greens, fennel
	Juice	Juice may be made and used, without adding sweeteners, from the following: fruits—any listed above in any combination desired; vegetables—any listed above in any combination desired
Day 3	Grape	All varieties of grape and raisin
	Rose	Strawberry, raspberry, blackberry, dewberry, loganberry, youngberry, boysenberry, rose hip
	Legume	Pea, black-eyed pea, dry bean, string bean, carob, soybean, lentil, licorice, peanut, alfalfa

	Flaxseed	Flaxseed
	Suidae	All pork products
	Arrowroot	Arrowroot
	Oil	Peanut, soy
	Sweetener	Carob syrup (use sparingly), clover honey (if honey not used on any other day)
	Tea	Alfalfa, rose hip
	Juice	Juice may be made and used, without adding sweeteners, from the following: fruits—any listed above in any combination desired; vegetables—any listed above in any combination desired
Day 4	Heath	Blueberry, huckleberry, cranberry, wintergreen
	May apple	May apple
	Papaw	Papaw, papaya, papain
	Composites	Lettuce, chicory, endive, escarole, artichoke, dandelion, sunflower seed, tarragon, oyster plant (salsify), celtuce
	Morning glory	Sweet potato (not yam)
	Laurel	Avocado, cinnamon, bay leaf, sassafras, cassia bud or bark
	Protea	Macadamia nut
	Beech	Chestnut
	Orchid	Vanilla
	Fungus	Mushroom, yeast (brewer's yeast, baker's yeast, and such)
	Salt-water fish	Sea herring, anchovy, cod, sea bass, sea trout, mackerel, tuna, swordfish, flounder, sole
	Spurge	Tapioca
	Oil	Avocado
	Tea	Sassafras, papaya
	Juice	Juice may be made and used, without adding sweeteners, from the following: fruits—any listed above in any combination desired; vegetables—any listed above in any combination desired
Day 5	Pineapple	Pineapple
	Gourd	Watermelon, cucumber, cantaloupe, pumpkin, squash (all varieties), other melons, zucchini, summer squash
	Purslane	Purslane, New Zealand spinach
	Mallow	Okra, cottonseed

	Cashew	Cashew, pistachio, mango
	Pedalium	Sesame
	Mollusca	Abalone, snail, squid, clam, mussel, oyster, scallop
	Crustacea	Crab, crayfish, lobster, prawn, shrimp
	Oil	Cottonseed, sesame
	Tea	Fenugreek
	Juice	Juice may be made and used, without adding sweeteners, from the following: fruits—any listed above in any combination desired; vegetables—any listed above in any combination desired
Day 6	Banana	Banana, plantain, arrowroot (Musa)
	Pomegranate	Pomegranate
	Ebony	Persimmon
	Palm	Coconut, date, date sugar, sago, palm cabbage
	Pepper	Black pepper, peppercorn
	Nutmeg	Nutmeg
	Beet	Beet, chard, spinach, lamb's-quarters
	Birch	Filbert, hazelnut
	Bird	Turkey, duck, pigeon, pheasant, and their eggs
	Oil	Coconut, fat from any bird listed above
	Sweetener	Date sugar, beet sugar (use sparingly)
	Juice	Juice may be made and used, without adding sweeteners, from the following: fruits—any listed above in any combination desired; vegetables—any listed above in any combination desired
Day 7	Plum	Plum, cherry, peach, apricot, nectarine, almond, wild cherry, small amounts of any natural dried fruit listed above
	Mustard	Mustard, turnip, radish, horseradish, watercress, cabbage, kraut, chinese cabbage, broccoli, cauliflower, brussels sprouts, collard, kale, kohlrabi, rutabaga
	Yam	Yam, chinese potato
	Brazil nut	Brazil nut
	Conifer	Pine nut
	Bovidae	Lamb
	Oil	Safflower

Sweetener	Buckwheat, safflower, and sage honey (if honey not used on any other day)
Tea	Safflower, maté
Juice	Juice may be made and used, without adding sweeteners, from the following: fruits—any listed above in any combination desired; vegetables—any listed above in any combination desired

Special tips for using the rotation diet

How to switch food families

The preceding pages have presented the food families and have given plans for four-day and seven-day diets. If you would like a food on a different day from where it has been indicated, you may switch the entire family to another day. When you have the food family on the day you prefer, leave it on that day so that the food is not eaten more often than prescribed.

Substitutes for common foods

Margarine: Use the oil of the day, mix in a blender with nuts and seasonings. This can be used to top vegetables.

Beverages: Use the spices of the day—mace, nutmeg, anise, cinnamon, clove—and brew as a tea; mix an equal amount of the tea with fruit juice. Serve iced or hot.

Egg: Use 8 ounces of dried apricots soaked until soft in 2 cups of water and mix in the blender. A generous tablespoon of this mixture is equal to one egg in a dough mixture. Another substitute is 1 cup of ground flaxseed boiled for three minutes in 3 cups of water. Stir constantly. Keep in closed jar in refrigerator. One tablespoon equals one egg. There are also commercial egg substitutes on the market.

Milk: Mix 2 ounces of almonds, pine nuts, or 1 teaspoon of sesame seeds with 1 teaspoon of honey and 1 cup of water in a blender for use in recipes. There are also commercial soy milk products on the market.

Salad dressings: Use ascorbic acid (vitamin C), 1 tablespoon to 1 cup of water, as a substitute for vinegar in salad dressings. Combine the vitamin C mixture, the oil of the day, salt, and spices of the day to give you a great variety of dressings. Avocado, tomato, onion, celery, and other vegetables and cheeses can be added as the day allows.

Purposeful violation of the diversified rotation diet

When a rotation is successfully established, it is possible occasionally to eat a single meal of multiple foods without respect to rotation. It is best to reserve this as a treat for special occasions once a month or so. Alcohol should not be used with this meal, as it will multiply by four the chances of a reaction occurring. When needed, a considerable degree of protection from maladaptive reactions to these special occasion meals can be achieved by the following, taken singly or as a total program:

1. One hour ahead of the meal take 4 grams of sodium ascorbate (vitamin C).
2. One hour ahead of the meal take five 350-milligram pancreatic-enzyme capsules or tablets. (Some do better by adding three to five 100-milligram bromelain tablets to this.)
3. One hour ahead of the meal take 5 to 15 grams of free amino acids.
4. Immediately ahead of the meal, take sublingually (under the tongue) 1,250 to 2,500 units of heparin. Heparin sublingually placed in this dosage can serve as a great protection against inflammatory allergic reactions. This can be

given ten to fifteen minutes before a meal; and, if a reaction to a meal occurs, it can be used immediately to help reduce the symptoms. It is easy for a person to carry heparin with him and have it readily available for sublingual use. This amount of heparin is considerably below the anticoagulant doses for which heparin has been placed on the market, but it does serve as a good anti-inflammatory agent at this level. Heparin can also be used as a protection against petrochemical hydrocarbons during unavoidable exposure to exhaust fumes. It is not wise to use these anti-inflammatory agents to try to ride through a chronic exposure where avoidance and spacing of contact can be arranged, but they do serve a valuable purpose in making life more comfortable when this is impossible.

5. With the meal, take 500 milligrams of pyridoxine, 100 to 500 milligrams of riboflavin, and 500 milligrams of pantothenic acid.
6. At the end of the meal, take one pancreatic-enzyme capsule or tablet. (Some do better by adding a 100-milligram bromelain tablet to this.)
7. Half an hour to an hour after the end of the meal, take one to five pancreatic-enzyme capsules or tablets. (Some do better by adding one or two 100-milligram bromelain tablets to this.)
8. Half an hour to an hour after the meal, take 10 to 20 grams of sodium bicarbonate or sodium and potassium bicarbonate (3:1 ratio).
9. If any symptoms develop after the meal, take 2,500 units of heparin sublingually. Also, the pancreatic enzymes and bicarbonate can be taken sooner than the thirty- to sixty-minute period if symptoms occur. A much more detailed discussion on the use of this type of nutrient therapy will be forthcoming in subsequent chapters.

Chemically contaminated food

Many foods inherently contain toxins that require detoxification by the liver or by other metabolic means, such as the operation of vitamin C or oxygenation. Molds producing toxins and/or occasioning maladaptive allergies or allergic-like reactions are frequent in foods. The widespread use of pesticides in recent years has added toxic residues to fruits, vegetables, and feed crops with resultant contamination of meat and milk, which adds to the burden of detoxification placed on the system. This, and the increase in potential maladaptive reactions, hastens the degenerative disease process. Efforts are being made to reduce levels of toxins in our foods and water supply, but some people are so sensitive and have such a low level of detoxifying ability that they must use nonchemically contaminated foods and water. Dr. Randolph and several others who have followed his lead have demonstrated the value of initially testing with nonchemically contaminated foods and then later selectively testing nonreactive foods contaminated with insecticides.[15,16] Dr. Mandell has demonstrated the value of sublingual provocative testing to determine maladaptive reactions to insecticide residues.

Summary

The latter part of the nineteenth century and the early part of the twentieth brought to medicine a significant array of ecologic facts that not only led to some valuable present-day health measures but also helped to develop the fields of bacteriology and allergy. Before the ecologic orientation had made its full contribution, however, such body-centered areas as pathology and pharmacology (drugs) were giving promise of rapid cure and/or quick symptomatic relief. The promise of such treatment methods tended to eclipse the significance of ecologic facts. Recently, a resurgence of interest in human ecology has been occurring due to the developing consciousness of how the ever-increasing pollution of our entire environment is adversely influencing man. Another factor causing this trend is the clinically demonstrated position that there is evidence to prove frequently eaten foods and commonly met chemicals are capable of adversely altering central-nervous-system functions.

The ecologic method of comprehensive environmental control provides for a specific period of avoidance of all possible incriminating substances. Such a program, in many cases, actually "turns off" by the fourth day the chronic physical or mental illness. The illness is turned back on by precipitating an acute reaction upon a single exposure to a food or chemical. In this way, induction evidence of symptom causes is clearly demonstrated; therefore, we can at least believe what we see. This evidence leads to the conclusion that the basic organic driving forces behind many chronic physical and mental illnesses are addictive reactions to frequently eaten foods and commonly met chemicals. After one has been exposed to all the ecologic facts presented in this book, a significant message should be obvious: Any food and/or chemical is capable of maintaining chronic physical and mental reactions in susceptible persons, and following a four- to seven-day period in which incriminating foods and chemicals are faithfully avoided results in clinical improvement in chronic symptoms. However, the sad truth is that we Americans are eating our foods with a frequency that is beyond our biological capacity to handle in a healthy way. After seeing hundreds of clinical cases, it has become increasingly clear to us that if people were taught to rotate their foods, many chronic physical and mental illnesses would be prevented. Not only can this rotation program provide a frequency contact that the human organism can metabolically handle and for which it was designed, it can also materially improve the nutritional state of each and every one of us due to the fact that we are contacting a desirably larger assortment of foods in a properly managed four-day rotation diet.

One can say that allergy and its counterpart, addiction, along with nutritional deficiency and infection are the building blocks from which chronic diseases are built. It matters not with which one of these we start; the others will soon follow. Of these three, the most important beginning point of many illnesses, as far as our clinical evidence reveals, is that of allergy-addiction, with nutritional deficiency and infection following closely.

It cannot be overemphasized that a four-or-more-day rotation of foods (especially symptom-incriminated foods) is of prime importance when attempting to control ecologically the allergic-addictive states. But it would certainly be wrong to conclude that a rotation diet alone is the cure-all of physical and mental illness. Nutrients in proper amounts and types can help prevent the majority of maladaptive reactions to foods and/or chemicals. Intravenous and oral administration of nutrients have been demonstrated clinically to be capable of preventing maladaptive allergic-addictive food and chemical reactions. Therefore, the ideal form of treatment combines both the ecological and the orthomolecular treatment methodologies. In order that we can begin to understand the fundamentals of the physical and mental disease process, let us now switch emphasis from food-chemical (ecological) management to nutritional orthomolecular management. An in-depth understanding of both of these important aspects of treatment is necessary.

Chapter 5

Supernutrition and the Orthomolecular Approach

Let us concede from the start that vitamins, minerals, trace elements, enzymes, and hormones (i.e., substances that normally occur in the human body) are not to be thought of as miraculous cure-alls. Rather, they are essential nutrients, and physical as well as mental illness will result when there is a deficiency of these chemicals in the human body. Sadly enough, even though this information is known in the scientific community, it is seldom considered as therapeutically important, especially by psychiatrists. Theoretically, psychiatrists as doctors should be interested in a nutritionally oriented differential diagnosis as much as any other physician should be. However, since it is known that the mind can influence body function, there has developed in psychiatry a bias favoring the expectation that the mind most often influences the body rather than the body influencing the mind. As a result of this attitude, when a psychiatrist observes a cluster of symptoms justifying a classic diagnosis such as neurosis or psychosis, she is then satisfied that the cause of the symptoms originates in the psyche, and any associated body symptoms are considered psychosomatic in origin. Once the psychiatrist makes her diagnosis of classifiable reactions, there is little chance she will consider any further need of a differential diagnosis relative to any of the patient's symptoms.

Differential diagnosis is a way to examine a patient other than by the usual psychiatric method considering clusters of symptoms.

It is a basic principle every doctor is taught early in his medical career. The method starts with a single symptom and includes all possibilities based on all known methods of diagnosis (i.e., history, physical examination, and laboratory diagnosis). The diagnosis must also take into consideration the ecologic factors of a patient's symptoms. It has been observed by M. B. Campbell, M.D., for example, that 69 percent of headaches are caused by ecologic factors, and yet there is probably less than a 1 percent chance that a doctor—even a specialist in neurology or psychiatry—will consider seriously the possibility of allergy (cerebral or otherwise) in his differential diagnosis.[17] Strong evidence indicates that for a majority of psychotics, ecologic factors as well as nutritional deficiencies materially influence their illness; yet there is little chance that these factors will be considered or examined for by specialists in psychiatry. If psychiatry had insisted on maintaining this method of diagnosis, then medicine as a whole would also have insisted on knowing the nutritional and ecological state of each patient. This failure to maintain an open differential diagnosis is perhaps psychiatry's greatest error in recent years. To test the possibility that nutritional deficiencies may relate to physical and/or emotional symptoms, no matter what the classic psychiatric diagnosis may be, I examined some two thousand patients of all diagnostic categories. The real breakthrough came when I demonstrated that maladaptive symptoms, ecologically diagnosed with prior testing of specific foods and chemicals, could actually be stopped by administering intravenously certain B vitamins and vitamin C. Now exciting evidence showed that certain nutrients could stop neurotic and psychotic reactions and that the results could be immediate.

The results of tests on three patients show this dramatically. The first test, given to a forty-four-year-old woman, indicated she had allergic reactions to cereal grains. After four days' avoidance, she was fed a test meal of wheat and immediately developed numbness in her throat, together with a feeling of choking and tightening of the neck muscles, hyperventilation, fatigue, headache, swollen eyelids and reddened eyes, a weakening of the legs so severe that she was unable to stand, flat affect, and an intense hot flash. Four days later she was fed a similar test meal, after receiving intravenously 7½ grams of vitamin C, 1,000 milligrams of pyridoxine (B_6), and the same amount of niacinimide (B_3). *No symptoms developed.* Two test meals, four days later, preceded by 3 grams of vitamin C, 1,000 milligrams of B_3, and 200 milligrams of B_6, administered orally, resulted in no symptoms after the first meal and only a minor hot flash after the second.

A thirty-nine-year-old woman was also tested for wheat after a four-day period of avoidance. Her symptoms included pounding of the heart, marked depression, loss of judgment, and loss of perspective about her present and future. Three weeks later, she was given two consecutive test meals, preceded by oral administration of 4 grams of vitamin C, 1,000 milligrams of B_3, 200 milligrams of B_6, 250 milligrams of thiamine (B_1), and 1 milligram of folic acid. The first test meal gave no symptoms; the second gave the patient a sense of loneliness.

A test meal of eggs made a twenty-seven-year-old man extremely agitated, nervous, and angry, and gave him the sensation of swelling in the head and neck. Three weeks later, after an egg food test preceded by 2,000 milligrams of B_3, 200 milligrams of B_6, 3,000 milligrams of C, 1 milligram of folic acid, and 60 milligrams of riboflavin (B_2), he suffered only the swelling feeling in his head and neck and none of the emotional symptoms.

The evidence demonstrates that in many cases it is possible to administer nutrients intravenously before feeding a test meal of a known maladaptive food reactor and to actually prevent the previously occurring reactions. Vitamins C, B_6, and B_3 have the most important value in preventing such maladaptive reactions. Vitamin C alone is effective for some, while B_6 alone is effective for others. In many cases, it is also possible to provide oral nutrients sufficiently far ahead of a meal for absorption to occur and thus prevent maladaptive food reactions. Testing indicated that if incriminated foods were given in enough consecutive meals, symptoms would develop in spite of nutrient therapy. Such evidence proved that nutrient therapy had to be combined with a diet based on a spaced rotation of food families. The most successful program included a four-day rotation diet combined with individualized appropriate nutrients given one and one-half hours ahead of each meal. However, in clinical practice, for convenience and best tolerance, the nutrients are given with the meals.

The following is an example of a portion of our clinical workup procedures (see also the following chart of symptoms and analyses). It involves a four-year-old infantile autistic boy. He presented symptoms of crying, temper tantrums, hyperactivity, insomnia, and short attention span and made gestures rather than spoke. He was not toilet trained. After four days of eating foods he seldom used, he was as calm as a normal child, which was a welcome contrast to his former hyperactivity, whirling around and screaming. Moreover, after the initial four-day avoidance period of commonly used foods, he became very cooperative as the testing proceeded, ate nearly everything offered him, made communicating sounds that were almost like words, and gave and received affection for the first time in many months. The cardinal symptoms of his illness emerged in response to test meals of specific foods that he frequently had at home.

Symptoms in Response to Deliberate Food Test of Single Foods

Food	*Reaction*
Soybean	Flatus
Pineapple	Weakness
Corn (fresh)	Agitated
Mature corn	Hyperactive, aggressive
Raisins	Anxious, very nervous
Honey	Very agitated. (Parents were surprised at his sudden change from being in a good mood to being extremely hyperactive and agitated. They said, "He has honey at home often.")
Bananas	Babbling
Cashews	Listless
Prunes	Severe diarrhea

Urine Amino Acid Analysis

Amino Acid	*Urine Results (mcm/24 hours)*		*Normal (mcm/24 hours)*
Phosphoserine	231+	(high)	21–90
Phosphoethanolamine	302+	(high)	26–101
Methionine sulfoxide	844+	(high)	150–650
Aspartic acid*	PT–***	(low)	11–80
Glutamic acid*	PT–	(low)	55–270
A-amino adipic acid**	431+	(high)	11–70
Valine	PT–	(low)	14–15
Cystine*	Absent	(low)	20–130
Cystathionine**	73+	(high)	8–55
Methionine**	148+	(high)	20–95
Phenylalanine	PT–	(low)	24–190
B-alanine	PT–	(low)	11–70
Hydroxylysine	Absent	(low)	10–13
1-me-Histidine	PT–	(low)	130–930
3-me-Histidine	PT–	(low)	30–180

* *Low amounts of aspartic acid, glutamic acid, and cystine suggest a vitamin B_6 utilization problem. Over 70 percent of our patients have such a disorder.*

** *High amounts of A-amino adipic acid, cystathionine, and methionine also suggest a B_6 utilization disorder. Morever, high levels of cystathionine and methionine in the urine have been shown to cause mental disorders.*

*** *PT = Present but deficient.*

Hair Analysis

Minerals and Trace Elements	*Results*		*Normal*
Calcium	2.0	(low)	25–57
Magnesium	0.1	(low)	3–7
Potassium	0.2	(low)	1–5
Copper	0.9	(low)	1.1–3.1
Zinc	3.0	(low)	13–20
Manganese	0.03	(low)	0.05–.17
Chromium	0.13	(high)	0.04–.07
Heavy Metals			
Cadmium	0.4	(high)	0.03–.1

Thyroid function was normal, but bacterial infections were present. *Progenitor cryptocides* was rated at 2½ on a scale of 0 to 4. Present were L forms, cogwheels, spent cells, misosomes, spicules, crystals, protoplasts, granular cells, and degenerate cells. A complete blood count revealed: Hematocrit, 39 (normal: 40 to 50); MCV, 79 (normal: 83 to 99), and Segmented, 67 (normal: 50 to 65).

The hair analysis involves two tablespoons of hair taken from the nape of the neck and sent to a laboratory. When properly interpreted, it provides the physician information about deficiencies in important minerals or excessive amounts of harmful toxic elements like lead or mercury. Figure 5.1 (see pages 66–69) is an example of a hair-analysis test accompanied by relevant mineral ratios and toxic metal levels. Doctor's Data, one company that performs these hair tests, also gives a good description of sources, dosages, and functions of each mineral in their Nutrient Mineral Level Chart.

The next example studies an eighteen-year-old schizophrenic with autistic symptoms since childhood. John was first noted to have retarded speech development at age four. The chief complaint at the time of examination at age eighteen was that there was a lag in central-nervous-system function. This included obsessional thinking, mood swings, compulsive gesturing, and hyperactivity.

The following chart shows symptoms and analysis from the clinical workup.

Symptoms in Response to Deliberate Food Test of Single Foods

Food	*Reaction*
Wheat	Sneezing, laughing, pacing
Corn	Pacing, irritable
Apple	Negativistic
Raisin	Sleepy and irritable
Cherries	Negativistic, hyperactive
Sweet potato	Hyperactive
Tomato	Nausea, anxiety, vomiting
Beets	Hyperactive
Black olives	Headache, which lasted two hours

Cane sugar	Negativistic, restless
Dates	Runny nose, hard to please
Milk	Talkative, hyperactive

Hair Analysis

Minerals	***Results***
Manganese	low
Lithium	low
Iron	low
Calcium	low
Zinc	low
Sodium	high
Potassium	high

A folic acid deficiency was measured. Bacterial infections were present. A dark-field microscopic examination of the blood revealed the microbe *Progenitor cryptocides* was present and rated at 2 on a scale of 0 to 4. Also present in the blood were cogwheels, target cells, motile rods, granular cells, and degenerate cells.

Figure 5.1 pictorially describes some hair analysis tests and nutrient levels.

A statement by John's mother

John weighed 9½ pounds at birth. For the first year, his development was normal except that he was very active and hard to hold. By the time he was nineteen months of age, he was rarely still during the day and frequently restless and unable to sleep at night. At three years of age, he resisted sitting even long enough to eat and would often eat on the run. His food habits were rigid. He mainly ate toast, crackers, milk, or soup. He greatly feared choking and ate only strained fruit, vegetables, and meat. After the toddler stage, he never seemed to have an appetite. Our concern grew over his

FIGURE 5.1

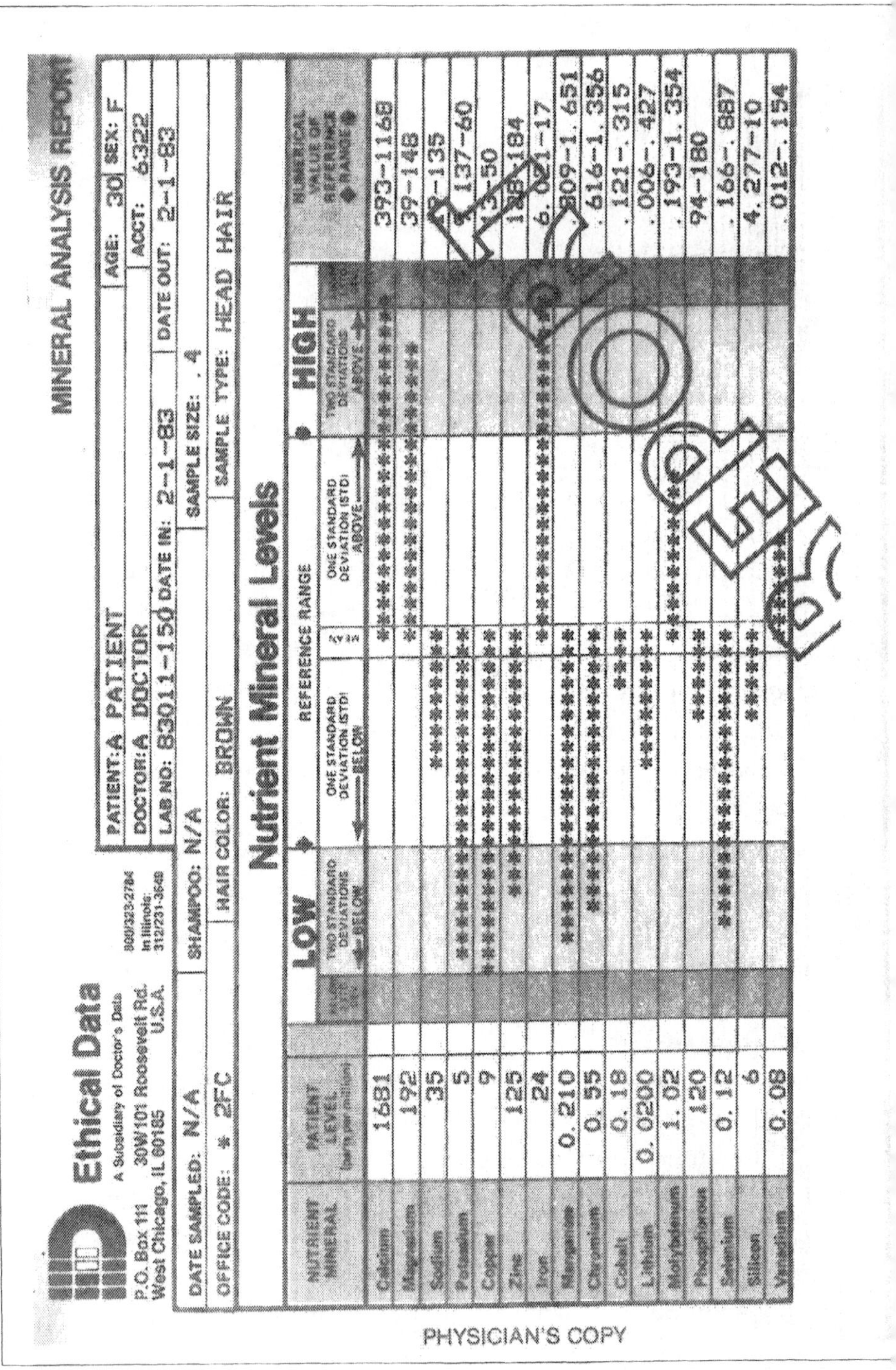

MINERAL ANALYSIS REPORT

Ethical Data
A Subsidiary of Doctor's Data
P.O. Box 111 30W101 Roosevelt Rd.
West Chicago, IL 60185 U.S.A.
800/323-2784
In Illinois: 312/231-3649

PATIENT: A PATIENT | AGE: 30 | SEX: F
DOCTOR: A DOCTOR | ACCT: 6322
LAB NO: 83011-150 | DATE IN: 2-1-83 | DATE OUT: 2-1-83
DATE SAMPLED: N/A | SHAMPOO: N/A | SAMPLE SIZE: .4
OFFICE CODE: * 2FC | HAIR COLOR: BROWN | SAMPLE TYPE: HEAD HAIR

Nutrient Mineral Levels

LOW — REFERENCE RANGE — HIGH

NUTRIENT MINERAL	PATIENT LEVEL (parts per million)	NUMERICAL VALUE OF REFERENCE RANGE
Calcium	1681	393-1168
Magnesium	192	39-148
Sodium	35	[illegible]-135
Potassium	5	[illegible] 137-60
Copper	9	13-50
Zinc	125	1[illegible]-184
Iron	24	6.021-17
Manganese	0.210	.[illegible]09-1.651
Chromium	0.55	.616-1.356
Cobalt	0.18	.121-.315
Lithium	0.0200	.006-.427
Molybdenum	1.02	.193-1.354
Phosphorous	120	94-180
Selenium	0.12	.166-.887
Silicon	6	4.277-10
Vanadium	0.08	.012-.154

PHYSICIAN'S COPY

SAMPLE

ADDITIONAL MINERAL LEVELS

Mineral	Level	Graph	Reference Range
Sulfur			
Strontium	3.000	*	.761-10
Barium	1.490	****	.338-3.503
Boron			
Gold	0.1300	*************	.105-.564
Silver	0.2500	*****	.064-.476
Tin	25.00	*********************	2.355-16
Antimony			
Tungsten	2.40	*****	.893-3.987
Zirconium	0.2000	*********	.126-.663

Toxic Mineral Levels

TOXIC MINERAL	PATIENT LEVEL (parts per million)	→ HIGH	ONE STANDARD DEVIATION ABOVE MEAN	TWO STANDARD DEVIATIONS ABOVE MEAN	MORE THAN TWO STANDARD DEVIATIONS ABOVE MEAN
Lead	12	*********	15		
Arsenic	3.10	*****	7		
Mercury	3.9	*************	2.5	******	
Cadmium	0.80	*********	1.0		
Aluminum	18	*******	30		
Nickel	1.60	********	2.2		
Beryllium	.0600	*******	10		

TOTAL TOXICS ************************************

RACE: SAMPLE CONDITION:

HAIR PREPARATIONS:

DRINKING WATER SOURCE:

Mineral Ratios

	LEVEL	REFERENCE RANGE
Ca/Mg	9	6.293-17
Ca/Zn	13.4	2.549-7.574
Ca/P	14.0	2.721-9.259
Ca/Fe	70.0	33-145
Ca/Mn	8005	470-2440
Mg/K	34.9	.977-10
Na/K	6.4	1.475-5.742
Zn/K	22.7	3.675-12
Zn/Cu	13.9	4.152-10
Cu/Fe	0.4	.904-5.772
Fe/Mn	114.3	6.725-36
Cu/Cd	11.2	37-201
Zn/Cd	156.3	289-1273
Se/Hg	0.03	.134-.583
Ca/Pb	140	78-348
P/Al	6.7	10-150

Lab Procedures According to ASETL Protocol John J. Errera, Director

Laboratory Work Performed By Doctor's Data Laboratories, Inc. CDC License No. 12104 IL License No. 13789

NUTRIENT MINERAL LEVEL CHART

	MINERAL	DAILY DOSAGE	AUGMENTING NUTRIENTS	ANTAGONISTS	RECOMMENDED SOURCES
A	Ca/Calcium	RDA: 800–1,400 mg SR: 1,000–2,000 mg Toxicity:	vitamins A, B_6, C, iron, magnesium, manganese, phosphorous, protein (especially lysine), silicon	lack of exercise, stress (excessive), too much oxalic and phytic acids, phosphorus (excessive), too much saturated fat in diet, Pb, Cd, Al, Mg, Fe	milk, cheese, molasses, yogurt almonds, 1 cup (325 mg) American cheese, 1 slice (200 mg) liver (beef), 1/4 lb. (500 mg)
B	Cr/Chromium	RDA: none stated SR: 100–300mcg Toxicity: not known	vitamin C	iron, stress	brewer's yeast, clams, corn oil, whole grain cereals, beer
C	Co/Cobalt	RDA: none stated SR: (as vitamin B_{12}) Toxicity: not known	iron	under investigation	lean muscle meats, organ meats
D	Cu/Copper	RDA: 2 mg SR: 2–4 mg Toxicity: 40 mg	cobalt, iron, zinc, molybdenum	zinc and manganese (high intakes), cadmum, oral contraceptives	legumes, nuts, organ meats, seafood (especially oysters), raisins, molasses, liver, avocado brazil nuts, 1 cup (4 mg) soybeans, 1 cup (2 mg)
E	Fe/Iron	RDA: 10–18 mg SR: 15–50 mg Toxicity: 100 mg	vitamins B_{12}, folic acid, C, calcium, cobalt, copper	coffee, excess phosphorus, tea, zinc or copper (excessive intake), manganese	blackstrap molasses, eggs, fish, organ meats, poultry, wheat germ, desiccated liver liver (beef), 1/4 lb. (200 mg) shredded wheat, 1 biscuit (30 mg)
F	Li/Lithium	RDA: none stated SR: 100–300mcg Toxicity: over 1.5 m Eq/L	vitamin E	under investigation	whole grains, seeds
G	Mg/Magnesium	RD: 300–350 mg SR: 300–350 mg Toxicity: 30,000 mg	vitamins B_6, C, D, calcium, phosphorus	protein, vitamin D, calcium (excessive intake), too much fat in diet, oral contraceptives	bran, honey, green vegetables, nuts, seafood, spinach, kelp tablets bran flakes, 1 cup (90 mg) peanuts (roasted w/skin), 1 cup (420 mg) tuna fish (canned), 1/2 lb. (150 mg)
H	Mn/Manganese	RDA: none stated SR: 1–50 mg Toxicity:	none	calcium/phosphorus (excessive intake), iron (excessive intake)	bananas, bran, celery, cereals, egg yolks, green leafy vegetables, legumes, liver, nuts, pineapples, whole grains
I	Mo/Molybdenum	RDA: none stated SR: 50–100mcg Toxicity:	none	copper sulfates, zinc, lead, methionine, vitamin B_{12}	whole grains, seeds, liver
J	P/Phosphorus	RDA: 800 mg SR: 800–1,000 mg Toxicity: not known	vitamins A, D, F calcium, iron, manganese	aluminum, iron, inorganic magnesium (antacids, milk of magnesia), white sugar (excessive)	eggs, fish, grains, glandular meats, meat, poultry, yellow cheese calf liver, 1/4 lb. (600 mg) milk yogurt, 1 cup (230 mg) eggs (cooked), 1 med. (110 mg)
K	K/Potassium	RDA: none stated SR: 100–300 mg Toxicity: not known Average daily intake: 1,950–5,850 mg	vitamin B_6, sodium	alcohol, coffee, cortisone, diuretics, laxatives, salt (excessive), sugar (excessive), stress	dates, figs, peaches, tomato juice, blackstrap molasses, peanuts, raisins, seafood apricots (dried), 1 cup (1,450 mg) bananas, 1 med. (500 mg) flounder, (baked), 1/4 1b. (650 mg) potatoes (baked), 1 med. (500 mg) sunflower seeds, 1 cup (900 mg)
L	Se/Selenium	RDA: none stated SR: 90–200mcg Toxicity: 500 mcg	vitamin E	mercury, cadmium, silver, arsenic, sulfates	fish, animal meats, whole grains, brown rice, pineapples
M	Si/Silicon	RDA: none stated SR: under investigation Toxicity: not known	high fiber diet	refined foods	plants (horsetail) and high fiber sources, celery, apple pectin
N	Na/Sodium	RDA: none stated SR: 100–300 mg Toxicity: 14,000 mg Average daily intake: 2,300–6,900 mg	vitamin D, potassium	chlorine/potassium (lack of)	salt, most foods and waters, including milk, cheese, seafood
O	V/Vanadium	RDA: none stated SR: 2–10 mg Toxicity: not known	not known	vitamins C and E, selenium	most water and foods, especially fats
P	Zn/Zinc	RDA: 15 mg SR: 20–100 mg Toxicity: not known	vitamins A and B, (high intake); calcium, copper, phosphorus	alcohol, stress, calcium or copper (high intake), phosphorus (lack of), phytic acid, oral contraceptives	brewer's yeast, liver, seafood, soybeans, spinach, sunflower seeds, mushrooms

TOXIC METAL LEVEL CHART

	TOXIC METAL	PROTECTIVE NUTRIENTS	SOURCES IN ENVIRONMENT	BODILY PARTS AFFECTED
Q	Al/Aluminum	none known	aluminum cooking utensils, antacids, foils, antiperspirants, aluminum containing baking powders, processed foods containing aluminum, soft water	stomach, bones, brain
R	As/Arsenic	iodine, selenium, calcium zinc, sulfur amino acids, Vitamin C	coal burning, pesticides, insecticides, herbicides, defoliants, metal smelting, manufacture of glass, mirrors, pesticides, insecticides, herbicides and defoliants	cells (cellular metabolism)
S	B/Beryllium	a specific not known—see Nutritional Therapies	(paints, colors, cosmetics)??? industrial exposure, mining, metal working, burning coal, copper processing	lungs, liver, kidney, heart
T	Cd/Cadmium	zinc, calcium, sulfur amino acids, vitamin C	cigarette smoke, oxide dusts, contaminated drinking water, galvanized pipes, paints, welding, pigments, contaminated shellfish from industrial seashores, teas, bone meal	renal cortex of kidney, heart and blood vessels, brain, appetite, smell centers
U	Pb/Lead	sulfur amino acids, vitamin C, E, calcium iron, zinc	leaded gas, lead based paint, newsprint and colored ads, hair dyes and rinses, dolomite, soft coal, leaded glass, pewter ware, pesticides, pencils, fertilizers, pottery, cosmetics, tobacco smoke, polluted air (average 35 mg/day in USA, higher in industrial areas and some cities)	bone, liver, kidney, pancreas, heart, brain, nervous system
V	Hg/Mercury	pectin, sulfur amino acids, vitamin C, selenium	manufacture and delivery of petroleum products, fungicides, fluorescent lamps, cosmetics, hair dyes, barometers, thermometers, amalgams in dentistry, salt water fish caught in contaminated waters	nervous system, appetite and pain center, cell membranes
W	Ni/Nickel	a specific not known—see Nutritional Therapies	nickel-cadmium batteries, jewelry, cosmetics, industrial exposure, hydrogenated oils, ceramic workers, cold waving (permanents), welding	point of exposure, skin ailments, lung cancer—industrial exposure. Nickel is essential at low levels. Some people are hypersensitive to nickel

BODILY FUNCTIONS FACILITATED	DEFICIENCY SYMPTOMS	THERAPEUTIC APPLICATIONS	OVERABUNDANCE
bone/tooth formation, blood clotting, heart rhythm, nerve tranquilization, nerve transmission, muscle growth and contraction, permeability of cell membranes	heart palpitations, insomnia, muscle cramps, nervousness, arm and leg numbness, tooth decay, osteoporosis, rickets, brittle fingernails, associated with gray hair	arthritis, aging symptoms (backache, bone pain, finger tremors), foot/leg cramps, insomnia, menstrual cramps, menopause problems, nervousness, overweight, premenstrual tension, rheumatism	most often indicates a deficiency, excess intake of dairy products or other calcium sources, environmental exposure
blood sugar level, glucose metabolism, circulatory system	atherosclerosis, glucose intolerance in diabetics, disturbed amino acid metabolism	diabetes, hypoglycemia, multiple pregnancies, protein-calorie malnutrition	cooking utensils, old stainless ware, environmental exposure
hemoglobin	iron deficiency anemia	iron deficiency anemia	excess ingestion with low protein intake
bone formation, hair and skin color, healing processes, hemoglobin and red blood cell formation, mental processes and emotional states	general weakness, impaired respiration, skin sores, diarrhea in infants, copper deficiency anemia, elevated cholesterol	copper deficiency anemia, baldness	copper water pipes, low zinc, excess dietary intake, check for exogenous source; i.e., swimming pool use
hemoglobin production, stress and disease resistance, growth in children	breathing difficulties, brittle nails, iron deficiency anemia (pale skin, fatigue), constipation, sore or inflammed tongue	alcoholism, anemia, colitis, menstrual problems, impaired absorption, blood loss	iron concentrations in water supply, excess dietary intake, environmental exposure
stable emotional states	manic-depressive disorders	manic depression	long term lithium therapy, environmental exposure
acid/alkaline balance, blood sugar metabolism (energy), metabolism (calcium and vitamin C), protein structuring (DNA, RNA)	confusion, disorientation, easily aroused anger, nervousness, rapid pulse, tremors	alcoholism, cholesterol (high), depression, heart conditions, M.I., kidney stones, nervousness, prostate troubles, sensitivity to noise, stomach acidity, tooth decay, overweight, protein-calorie malnutrition	most often indicates a deficiency, environmental exposure
enzyme activation, reproduction and growth, sex hormone production, tissue respiration, vitamin B, metabolism, vitamin E utilization, fat and carbohydrate metabolism	ataxia (muscle coordination failure), dizziness, ear noises, loss of hearing, abnormal carbohydrate and fatty acid metabolism, allergies, joint and back problems, metabolism	allergies, asthma, diabetes, fatigue	excess dietary intake, well water, environmental exposure (fumes from welding, soldering)
liver function, kidney function, blood, copper and iron metabolism	none known	copper deficiency anemia, gout	excess dietary intake, Cu deficiency, environmental exposure
bone/tooth formation, cell growth and repair, energy production, heart muscle contraction, kidney function, metabolism (calcium, sugar), nerve and muscle activity, vitamin utilization	appetite loss, fatigue, irregular breathing, nervous disorders, overweight, weight loss	arthritis, stunted growth in children, stress, tooth and gum disorders	lack of dietary calcium, excess intake of beef, soft drinks, most processed foods
heartbeat, rapid growth, muscle contraction, nerve tranquilization, kidneys, blood	acne, continous thirst, dry skin, constipation, general weakness, insomnia, muscle damage, nervousness, slow irregular heartbeat, weak reflexes	acne, alcoholism, allergies, burns, colic in infants, diabetes, high blood pressure heart disease (angina pectoris, congestive heart failure, myocardial infarction)	may indicate deficiency, check Na/K ratio
membrane integrity, pancreatic function (possible increased resistance to cancer), vitamin E utilization	mercury toxicity, pancreatic insufficiency, cardiac toxicity of drugs, aging pigment, peroxidation of fats, blood hemolytic problems, muscle wasting	cancer, mercury toxicity	environmental exposure, such as selenium in dandruff shampoos
bone calcification, skin, aorta, connective tissue, thymus	bone decalcification, tendonitis, cardiovascular disease	rapid aging, abnorma skeletal formation, atherosclerosis	silicon injections and implants, environmental exposure
normal cellular fluid level, proper muscle contraction, blood, lymph system	appetite loss, intestinal gas, muscle shrinkage, vomiting, weight loss	dehydration, fever, heat stroke	excess dietary intake, poor elimination, check for exogenous source
growth, reroduction, teeth, skeletal, liver, lipids, cholesterol	unknown in man. Rats: reduced growth, increased dental caries, triglycerides, blood and bone iron, altered hematocrit, cholesterol, phospholipids	elevated triglycerides, cholesterol, dental caries	usually airborne, contaminated water and food
burn and wound healing, carbohydrate digestion, prostate gland function, reproductive organ growth and development, sex organ growth and maturity, vitamin B_6, phosphorus and protein metabolism	fatigue, decreased taste acuity, night blindness, flatulence, poor appetite, delayed sexual maturity, prolonged wound healing, retarded growth, sterility	alcoholism, atherosclerosis, baldness, cirrhosis, diabetes, internal and external wound and injury healing, high cholesterol (eliminates deposits), infertility, impotency, prostate problems	may indicate deficiency, low intake of copper rich foods, excess dietary intake, environmental exposure (hair shampoos, sprays)

INTERFERES WITH BODILY FUNCTIONS	TOXICITY SYMPTOMS	NUTRITIONAL THERAPIES
irritating to gut, affects bone formation, brain convulses (high concentrations)	gastrointestinal irritation, colic, rickets, convulsions	garlic,eggs, beans, high sulfur amino acid supplements, vitamin C
metabolic inhibitor (reduces energy production efficiency), cellular and enzyme poison	fatigue, low vitality, listlessness, loss of pain sensation, loss of body hair, skin color changes (dark spots), gastroenteritis	garlic, eggs, beans, high sulfur amino acid supplements, vitamin C, proper iodine and selenium levels in diet
enzyme inhibitor including ATP, DNA, and several hepatic enzymes; cell death in all tissues	dyspnea, weight loss, cough, fatigue, chest pain, anorexia, weakness	unknown
heart and blood vessel structure (hypertension), (hypotension), kidneys, blocks appetite and smell centers, calcium metabolism	hypertension, hypotension, kidney damage, loss of sense of smell, decreased appetite	garlic, eggs, beans, high sulfur amino acid supplements, vitamin C, high calcium levels in diet
enzyme poison, osteoblast production, blood formation, blocks enzymes at cell level	weakness, listlessness, fatigue, pallor, abdominal discomfort, constipation, long-term memory, sophisticated thought	garlic, eggs, beans, high sulfur amino acid supplements, vitamin C, maintain high calcium, iron, and vitamin E in diet
destroys cells, blocks transport of sugars (energy at cell level), and increases permeability of potassium	loss of appetite and weight, severe emotional disturbances, tremors, blood changes, inflammation of gums, chewing and swallowing difficulties, loss of sense of pain, convulsions	garlic, eggs, beans, high amino acid supplements (especially cystine), vitamin C, selenium
DNA (trace amounts are necessary for several liver dehydrogenous enzymes, glutamate, GOT, GPT, etc.)	cancer, contact dermatitis, skin rashes, gingivitis, stomatitis, dizziness	garlic, eggs, beans, sulfhydryl amino acids, pectin, ascorbic acid, tocopherols

delayed speech. He could say a few words but rarely spoke. Sometimes he seemed deaf. Other times his hearing seemed hyperacute, and he would put his hands over his ears. He communicated his wants mainly by taking an adult's hand and leading him.

At an early age, he began twirling objects such as pan lids and even garbage can lids. Between three and four years of age, he began drawing the phases of the moon and traffic signs. He seemed fascinated by stop signs and would say "stop sign" over and over.

Shortly before he was five years of age, he was admitted to the diagnostic nursery associated with a medical school. He was started on a drug, Mellaril®. Now he would speak in short sentences, but it still seemed a painful effort. He preferred to work and play alone, ignoring the other children.

On several occasions, he had severe panic reactions for no apparent reason. When he was six years old, he bolted out of a department store into the street, obviously terrified, and refused for years to go into this store.

After three years at the diagnostic nursery, we were told to place him in a public school for children with disabilities. He had stayed longer at the nursery than any other child and was an enigma to them. The next few years were a traumatic time for both my child and me. Fortunately, after two years, a church school established a special education class, and John was one of the first admitted.

With the onset of puberty, he grew very rapidly and began to seem exhausted much of the time. He had continual respiratory infections, some of which were quite severe. He was irritable and began to have bizarre hand movements, facial grimaces, and a purposeless laugh. He developed severe hay fever and insomnia.

In February 1976, when John was eighteen years of age, he started on Dr. Philpott's orthomolecular-ecologic regime. From the third day of fasting, we began to notice a change. John began to sleep soundly and has continued to do so. He doesn't need any drugs. Even before the food testing was over, he was obviously much more alert and was speaking with less effort. Since being on the rotation diet and nutritional supplements prescribed, he has continued to improve remarkably. He is calm and feels well. The facial grimaces, hand movements, and purposeless laugh gradually subsided over about six months of time. His skin (acne) has improved and he has had no more infections of any kind. His hay fever has subsided. He has developed interest in many new areas and has even acquired a sense of humor. He is eager to go to school and is making steady progress academically and socially in a private school with students of normal intelligence. He particularly enjoys gymnastics at school. His increasing self-confidence is evident. His growing emotional maturity is a joy to behold.[18]

Format for supernutrition

Supernutrition is based on the idea that an ideal environment for each cell of our body includes not only an ample supply of water and oxygen and a suitable ambient temperature but also a team of about forty nutrients, all of which must be combined in just the right proportions in order to work together toward the ideal of perfect health. Thus, it is clear that adding any one nutrient to a person's diet as a supplement can bring no favorable result unless the diet contains adequate amounts of all the other nutrients. A list of these vitamins, minerals, and amino acids, and of the foods high in them, can be found in the appendix, which contains much technical information not covered in the main body of this book.

Obviously, the cells usually have to put up with environments that fall short of the ideal. And even if there were a perfect assortment of nutrients supplied to the body, the digestion, absorption, and transportation of these nutrients is not an automatic process that always takes place with perfection. This, of course, implies that if any link in the biochemical chain is weak or missing, the cells will be inadequately supplied, and ill health will quickly follow. The weak link might be something like an iron or calcium deficiency, a tyrosine (amino acid) deficiency, a vitamin B_6 deficiency, an improper absorption or digestion of these nutrients, deficiency of a trace mineral like selenium or molybdenum, and so on. The result of any of these deficiencies, plus the possibility of an almost infinite number of other deficiencies, is always the same: an impoverished biochemical environment, which inevitably leads to functional impairment.

Another roadblock on the pathway toward perfect health and an optimum supply of nutrients to all our cells is the fact that nutritional needs are distinctively different for each and every person alive. Hence, there can be no general program that everyone can or must follow. Each person's biochemical uniqueness must be taken into account. We cannot, for example, safely assume that furnishing a high-quality, protein-rich diet will provide adequate amounts of all the essential amino acids necessary for optimum health. There are numerous digestive enzymes that break down protein into amino acids, some of which in certain people might be functioning well and in others not functioning at all. Obviously, if the former is the case, there will be an adequate supply of amino acids in the blood; if the latter is true, this supply will be deficient. For vitamins as well as minerals and trace elements, each individual's unique need levels are even more distinctive. In fact, vitamin-tolerance levels may vary as much as a thousandfold among patients in the clinic.

It becomes obvious in light of the preceding observations that the field of nutrition is no playground for amateurs. Indeed, if supernutrition is to be used in the battle against disease, experts must be engaged in the undertaking. However, there are certain limited, preventive, and self-diagnostic measures an individual can usefully take; these are discussed in chapter 9.

The goal of supernutrition is optimum health for each cell of the body, and there is substantial evidence that this goal can be attained or closely approached. There may be cells, tissues, or organs that are so defective—because of genetic inheritance, environmental abuse, malnutrition, and so on—that they cannot be reached by supernutritional methods, but this should not be assumed to be true until serious attempts toward this goal prove otherwise.

Linus Pauling, Ph.D., defines orthomolecular medicine as that discipline which "varies the concentrations of substances (i.e., vitamins, minerals, trace elements, amino acids, hormones, enzymes, and so on) normally present in the human body in the treatment of disease and, in particular, mental disease. The methods," he continues, "principally used now for treating patients with mental disease are psychotherapy (psychoanalysis and related efforts to provide insight and to decrease environmental stress), chemotherapy (mainly with the use of powerful synthetic drugs, such as chlorpromazine, or powerful natural products from plants, such as reserpine), and convulsive shock therapy (electroconvulsive therapy, insulin coma therapy, pentylenetetrazol shock therapy). I have reached the conclusion that another general method of treatment, which may be called orthomolecular therapy, may be found to be of great value, and may turn out to be the best method of treatment for many patients."[19]

Orthomolecular physicians insist that the battle against disease, and, in particular, mental disease, should always begin with weapons—nutrients—that are most similar to nature's own biological weapons. For if we are sick in any way, the orthomolecular view is that the cells of our bodies are ailing because they are being inadequately provisioned with the nutrients they need for proper metabolism and health. We have already pointed out that should a cell become deficient in any one or group of nutrients its entire function will be seriously impaired. And if you multiply one deranged cell by a few hundred million, then tissues and organs, even the brain, are affected, and one experiences what modern medicine calls degenerative disease. The brain, for example, is an organ composed of millions of cells. It perceives, thinks, feels, orders behavior, and has memory. When its metabolism becomes disordered due to nutritional deficiencies—and this is usually the case in a majority of the patients at our clinic—the brain expresses this disorder by changes in perception of one or more of the senses or in thinking (i.e., illusions, hallucinations, delusions). As a result of an altered perception of sense and reason, one's behavior and mood are often dramatically changed for the worse.

The "team" of necessary nutrients are specific chemicals that can be found in varying amounts in each one of us. Enzymes catalyze or speed up the reactions in the body by which our food is broken down into these basic nutrients, which are required for structural development and for the production of energy. If a person with specific individual requirements for these nutrients lives on a diet which contains less than his requirements, in time he will develop a deficiency state which produces its characteristic syndrome. The reasons for the varying ranges in nutrient needs among individuals is relatively unknown, but there is some evidence that, for example, a B_3 deficiency maintained for a prolonged period of time can lead to a permanent dependency. Around 1935, it was discovered that dogs maintained on a pellagra-producing diet (a totally B_3-deficient diet) required very large dosages (megadosages) of vitamin B_3 in order to keep them free of pellagra (manifested by dermatitis, gastrointestinal disorders, and central nervous symptoms). The researchers were amazed to find that some adult pellagrins required maintenance dosages of 600 milligrams or larger of vitamin B_3 to keep them free of pellagra. This amount is over sixty times as high as that considered necessary by many nutritionists to prevent pellagra. Further evidence for deficiency-induced dependence comes to us from prisoners of war kept in Japanese prison camps for over forty-four months. A number of Canadian soldiers maintained on starvation diets for this long period suffered from a variety of nutrient deficiencies. These soldiers have remained chronically ill since their imprisonment. The exceptions are a dozen veterans, all once as seriously ill as the rest, who were given specific nutrients in megadosages. All these men improved significantly and have remained well since. When one man tried going off his nutrient therapy, his original symptoms developed almost immediately. Convinced by his experiential evidence, he has remained on the nutrient program prescribed for him by an orthomolecular physician.

Mental illness, and an assortment of physical diseases, can result from a low concentration in the brain of any one of the following vitamins: thiamine (B_1), niacin (B_3), pyridoxine (B_6), hydroxocobalamin (B_{12}), pantothenic acid, folic acid, and ascorbic acid (C). Mental function and behavior can, of course, be affected by changes in the concentration in the brain of other nutrients, but for now let us closely examine some of the clinical evidence concerning these especially significant vitamins.

Vitamin B_1 deficiency causes loss of appetite generated by cell malnutrition in the hypothalamus. Other symptoms can include irritability, depression, confusion, loss of memory, inability to concentrate, fear of impending doom, and a rather acute sensitivity to noise. All of these symptoms disappear when thiamine is administered in proper megadosages.[20]

Vitamin B_3 deficiency results in pellagra. The earliest symptoms are anxiety, depression, chronic fatigue, and vague somatic complaints.[21] Investigators Frostig and Spies classified sixty patients as suffering from pellagra. All the patients manifested hyperactivity, hyperesthesia, depression, fatigue, apprehension, and insomnia, and some suffered with chronic headaches. Clinically speaking, the requirement of vitamin B_3 for proper functioning of the brain is well known. The psychosis of pellagra, as well as the other manifestations of this deficiency disease, is prevented by the intake of a small amount of niacin (20 milligrams a day). However, once a deficiency has been established, this dosage must be increased significantly. Acute cases of pellagra quickly respond to 1 to 2 grams of niacin a day, but the chronic cases respond more slowly and often have to double this dosage. In 1939, Cleckley, Sydenstricker, and Geeslin reported the successful treatment of nineteen patients with severe psychiatric symptoms with niacin, and in 1941, Sydenstricker and Cleckley reported similarly successful treatment of twenty-nine patients with niacin. In both studies, moderately large dosages of niacin (0.3 to 1.5 grams a day) were given. In 1964, Hoffer and Osmond reported that a ten-year, double-blind study of patients using niacin and those not using the vitamin demonstrated that 75 percent of those using the nutrient did not require hospitalization during this period, while only 36 percent of the comparison group who had not received niacin did not require hospitalization.

Nicotinamide-adenine dinucleotide (NAD) is an active enzyme that is required for the proper function of vital areas of the brain. In schizophrenia, there appears to be a failure to deliver enough NAD to the brain. Vitamin B_3 is required for the transformation of tryptophan, an amino acid, into NAD. If there is a niacin deficiency, this necessary transformation of tryptophan into NAD is inhibited, and there is not only a NAD deficiency established but also an overload of tryptophan in the brain's chemistry. Tryptophan is considered to be one of the most toxic of all the amino acids. An overload of it in the brain can be very harmful, especially if it is not properly converted into NAD because it can cause undesirable perceptual and mood changes. If there is a B_3 deficiency, for whatever reason, the consequent NAD deficiency will lead to ever-increasing trytophan overload unless and until the proper levels of B_3 are given.

Pyridoxine, or vitamin B_6, is used in the treatment of cerebral allergies by many orthomolecular physicians. There is clinical evidence that pyridoxine is involved in the tryptophan-niacin metabolism previously explained. Moreover, B_6 is a precursor to over sixty enzyme reactions, is necessary for the proper metabolism of all the amino acids, and is required for the maintenance of a stable immunologic system. A substance called kryptopyrrole (KP), also called the "mauve factor," has been shown to be abnormally present in the urine of psychiatric patients, especially schizophrenics, and to deplete the system of B_6 and zinc.[22] Patients with too much KP (i.e., over 20 milligrams per 100 milliliters of blood) must be given megadoses of pyridoxine as well as zinc and usually respond favorably to these nutrient supplements. Moreover, since B_6 is related to NAD, any deficiency in this area, along with the corresponding tryptophan overload, is easily corrected with the proper B_6 and B_3 supplementation therapy.

A higher incidence of B_{12} deficiencies has been discovered in mental patients than in the general population. Symptoms resulting from B_{12} deficiency range from poor concentration to stuporous depression, severe agitation, and hallucinations. Pernicious anemia is a better-known symptom of this vitamin deficiency. Edwin and his associates have reported that the amount of vitamin B_{12} in the serum of every patient over thirty years old admitted to a mental hospital in Norway during a period of one year clearly demonstrated a 15.4 percent pathologically low concentration of the nutrient. H. L. Newbold, M.D., suggests that when the serum B_{12} level is below 200 micrograms per milliliter of blood, the patients should be routinely given at least monthly—if not weekly—injections of hydroxocobalamin at 1,000 micrograms per milliliter the remainder of their lives.[23] Certainly, this is good advice in view of the possible consequences of demyelination of the spinal cord and the brain itself in states where the serum B_{12} is low.

Volunteers fed a diet that was low in pantothenic acid very quickly became emotionally upset, irritable, quarrelsome, sullen, depressed, and dizzy. Roger J. Williams, Ph.D., discovered that both animals and humans could withstand more stress, physical and emotional, after receiving large dosages of pantothenic acid.[24] This is almost certainly due to the fact that this nutrient supports the adrenal gland, which handles physical as well as emotional stress via hormone regulation. Williams has also discovered that the wide variance observed in reactions of his subjects indicates that specific requirements of pantothenic acid may vary greatly.

Patients who are allergic to wheat gluten are usually low in blood histamine. C. C. Pfeiffer has clinically observed that this type of patient is not only low in blood histamine, but usually is high in serum copper and low in folic acid.[25] These patients are normally overstimulated, paranoid, and hallucinatory and respond well to niacin, B_{12}, and folic acid (2 milligrams daily). Folic acid in conjunction with weekly B_{12} shots raises the blood histamine, at the same time lowering the degree of psychopathology.

It was reported as far back as 1942 by M. K. Horwitt[26] and by later investigators that schizophrenic patients receiving the usual dietary amounts of vitamin C had considerably lower concentrations of this nutrient in their blood than people in good health. A very important controlled trial of vitamin C in chronic psychiatric patients was reported in 1963 by G. Milner.[27] The double-blind study was made with forty chronic male patients: thirty-four had schizophrenia, four had manic-depressive psychosis, and two had general paresis. Twenty of the patients, selected at random, were given 1,000 milligrams of vitamin C a day for three weeks; the rest of the group received a placebo. The patients were tested with the Minnesota Multiphasic Personality Inventory (MMPI) and the Wittenborn Psychiatric Rating Scales (WPRS) before and after the trial. Milner concluded that statistically significant improvement in the depressive, manic, and paranoid symptoms-complexes, together with an improvement in overall personality functioning, was obtained following saturation with ascorbic acid. He went on to suggest that many chronic psychiatric patients would benefit from the administration of ascorbic acid.

In another test of schizophrenic patients, discussed in detail in chapter 9, Linus Pauling concluded, "I have no doubt that many schizophrenic patients would benefit from an increased intake of ascorbic acid."[28] Obviously, this must be true when one considers the fact that in some schizophrenics, one can give as high as 40 grams per day before it spills into the patient's urine. This same occurrence happens when a nonschizophrenic individual contracts a severe virus infection and is given vitamin C in large doses. Megadoses of the nutrient can be given before a urine spillage is noticed. The relationships existing between vitamin C, infections, and mental illness will be discussed in detail later on, but for now, let us concede that clinical double-blind studies have proven that vitamin C is beneficial not only to physical but to mental health.

Some important minerals deserve mention. Potassium, for example, can be related to mental health. Symptoms of extreme fatigue, indifference, muscle weakness, and a lack of feeling were manifested by healthy volunteers who were fed a potassium-deficient diet.[29] These symptoms disappeared following administration of 10 grams of potassium chloride. Potassium is also an essential mineral present in intracellular fluid. It is necessary for proper growth and nerve function and is needed for certain enzyme reactions and synthesis of muscle protein. Potassium deficiencies can be caused by alcohol, coffee, and excessive use of salt and sugar. Many patients taking diuretics run into trouble with potassium deficiencies. They should always attempt to eat foods naturally rich in the mineral, such as oranges, bananas, or freshly prepared vegetables.

Calcium is the most abundant mineral in the body. Ninety-nine percent of calcium utilized by the body is deposited in bones and teeth. The remainder, located in the soft tissues, performs a number of necessary functions. Calcium aids in muscle contraction, including heartbeat, and in blood clotting and the transmission of neuromotor impulses. Symptoms of calcium deficiency are muscular irritability, softening of the bones, especially serious in the aged, and rickets in children. Since very large dosages of vitamin C can chelate calcium out of the body, it is important to supplement the diet with this most important mineral when vitamin C therapy is indicated. Moreover, calcium will not function properly unless magnesium, phosphorus, vitamins A and D, proteins, and a normal pH (or a normal acid-base) environment are present.

Magnesium is essential in metabolic processes, activating enzymes, regulating the body's pH, assisting in neuromuscular contraction, protein synthesis, and utilization of vitamins C, E, and the B-complex. A diet very high in calcium necessitates a dietary increase of magnesium; also, a high alcohol intake can lead to magnesium deficiency. Its deficiency is serious and can cause depression, irritability, tremors, irregular heartbeat, cirrhosis of the liver, and hardening of the arteries. Parenthetically, magnesium supplementation will be required for those who take large amounts of vitamin B_1. Williams has reported paranoia as a symptom of severe magnesium deficiency. The paranoia disappeared when magnesium was given.[30]

Phosphorus functions with calcium and is present in every human cell. It is essential to the digestion of niacin and riboflavin. Excesses of this mineral can result in a loss of calcium. Eighty percent of the body's phosphorus levels are used for bones and teeth in combination with calcium. Phosphorus also bonds itself with nicotonic acid to carry on other physiological processes. Since phosphorus combines with other substances in most foods, it is somewhat difficult to sustain a phosphorus deficiency.

Normally found in all human tissues, zinc is essential for the synthesis of protein and the action of more than thirty enzymes. As mentioned earlier, it is related to KP (kryptopyrrole) manifestations. It is needed in trace amounts for proper function of the B vitamins, certain enzyme reactions, and tissue respiration. Vitamin A must be present for zinc to be absorbed. Zinc deficiency affects taste and smell and may cause apathy, flat emotional responses, and lethargy. Other zinc deficiency-related problems are retardation of growth (as a result of unpalatability of food), delayed wound healing, interrupted reproduction, diminished learning capacity, and general diminishment of proper protein and carbohydrate metabolism. Furthermore, zinc is related to sexual function, and impotent males deficient in this particular mineral require many months of zinc supplementation before normal potency is regained. The human skin contains about 20 percent of all the body's zinc. Zinc-deficient fingernails and toenails will be brittle and show opaque white spots on them. When the skin is deficient of this important mineral, stretch marks appear over hips, thighs, abdomen, breasts, and shoulders. According to Pfeiffer, zinc deficiency is likely to appear during the following conditions: pregnancy, rapid growth years, puberty, severe stress conditions, serious illness, and birth-control medication, which elevates copper levels, resulting in a diminishment of zinc.

Iron is probably the best known of all the minerals. Its major functions are in the production of hemoglobin in blood and myoglobin in muscle tissue. An iron deficiency will cause an insufficiency of hemoglobin and resultant anemia. Iron deficiency can result from hemorrhage or simply poor assimilation. It is noteworthy to mention that coffee and tea interfere with proper iron absorption.

Manganese is essential in trace amounts as an enzyme activator. It is also essential for nerve and brain function. It is required for the synthesis of acetylcholine, which is a neurotransmitter, and a deficiency may be casually connected with diabetes mellitus, as diabetics appear to have low manganese levels in their bodies. Zinc and manganese work together to reduce excess copper in the body. Animals deficient in manganese demonstrate retarded growth, hyperactivity, uncoordinated movements, and poor equilibrium.

Copper is considered by some to be primarily toxic, but it does in fact play an important role in iron absorption, functioning of vitamin C, synthesis of phospholipids, bone formation, RNA production, and formation of red blood cells. Certain conditions, such as pregnancy or the use of birth-control pills, cause an elevation in serum (blood) copper. Excess copper levels have been recorded frequently in different groups of schizophrenics. Interestingly enough, copper and zinc are biologically antagonistic toward each other; therefore, in animal studies using either or both of these metals, it has been shown that any dietary excess of one will automatically lead to a depletion of the other. Any excessive ingestion of copper will cause health problems. The common use of copper pipes in our home plumbing systems adds to the possibility of such an excessive ingestion due to the leaching of the mineral into drinking water. It is a good idea to avoid drinking the first water that comes from the tap of a copper plumbing system. Let it run for a few minutes in order to reduce the copper levels found in the water that has been sitting in the pipes for a long time.

Sodium is both essential and abundant and is present in almost every food. In extracellular fluid, sodium functions with potassium to keep blood minerals soluble and to aid in digestion. Too much sodium should be avoided since an excess can damage the heart and the kidneys. Patients with Addison's disease or a weakened adrenal system, however, can experience severe fatigue partly because of the lack of a sodium-retention hormone secreted by the adrenal gland. Also, sodium deficiency has become an increasingly more serious problem in recent years because of the widespread use of diuretic drugs.

Chromium must be present in order for the insulin hormone of the pancreas to function properly and supply glucose (blood sugar) to every cell of the body. As further research develops, this mineral will receive intensive investigation as a treatment possibility for diabetes mellitus and other blood-sugar-related disorders.

Selenium is not toxic in amounts less than 5 milligrams and is an absolutely essential trace mineral. It greatly increases the efficacy of vitamin E and works as its partner as an antioxidant. It also helps to maintain tissue elasticity and prevent chromosome breakage. Moreover, it protects us against toxic levels of trace poisons such as cadmium and mercury. It is interesting to note that when selenium intake has been low, the cancer rate has been high.

Iodine in trace amounts is necessary for proper thyroid function and metabolism, as it is a component of the thyroid hormone thyroxine. Although large doses of iodine are highly toxic, deficiencies are more common and may result in goiter or hypothyroidism. When this happens at a young age, both physical and mental development is stunted, producing cretinism and feeblemindedness. Iodine is regularly added to table salt and is abundantly present in seafood.

The concept that some minerals as well as vitamins, now called micronutrients, may be deficient in some types of physical and mental illness, and in particular in schizophrenia, is not entirely new. What is new is the fact that orthomolecular physicians are using biochemical analysis in order to treat these specific deficiencies and finding success in doing so. It is always important to remember that supernutrition is arranged according to the findings in each individual's case. Consequently, there can be no general program appropriate for everyone, and only a very rough outline of specific dosages of these nutrients can be given.

Niacin or niacinamide should not exceed 1,000 milligrams three times a day; half the amount or less is preferable. The dosage of every vitamin must be tailored to the severity of the individual allergic-addictive reactions of each patient. Vitamin C should be kept below the level causing diarrhea. A reasonable dose would be 6, 8, or 10 grams for a twenty-four-hour period. These dosages should be given in three to four equal amounts. Some people can tolerate sodium ascorbate better than ascorbic acid. Either form of vitamin C is effective. It should be pointed out that when treating opportunist, infectious microbes, the dosages of vitamin C can be raised. Intravenous use of the nutrient is very effective in this respect. Some physicians give as much as 50 to 150 grams intravenously over a period of twenty-four hours in cases of extremely resistant infectious invasion. Such dosages should be given only under direct medical supervision.

The range of vitamin B_6 should be from a minimum of 50 milligrams three times a day to a maximum of 500 milligrams three times a day. When using dosages as much as 1,000 milligrams three times a day, numbness of the hands and feet have been reported. Folic acid is given at 400 micrograms to 1 milligram three times a day. No side effects have been noted. However, folic acid should not be given by itself in a B_{12}-deficient patient. B_{12} deficiency must be indicated by prior testing. Vitamin B_{12} is not routinely given, but when given orally, 1,000 micrograms three times a day is sufficient. No adverse side effects are known from this dosage. If vitamin B_{12} levels are abnormally low, 1,000 micrograms of hydroxocobalamin two to three times a week is given intramuscularly.

Vitamins B_1, B_2, B_5, and B_6 can range in dosages from 50 milligrams two to three times a day to 500 milligrams three times a day. Pantothenic acid (B_5) is given for its supportive as well as stimulating value for adrenal function and is used empirically in this respect. Vitamin E (400 units three times a day) is used empirically for its improvement of fat metabolism and its detoxifying values. The wheat-allergic patient should not use vitamin E from wheat-germ oil, but a synthetic form. It is important to note that vitamins B_6 and B_2 should be given together in order to maintain balanced nutrition. Large dosages of B_6 are thought to produce a relative riboflavin deficiency; in order to avoid this possibility, it is sometimes best to give both vitamins in equal amounts.

Vitamins A and D are also given empirically. Carl Reich, M.D., reports A and D as being useful in asthma.[31] It would be expected, therefore, to be useful in cerebral allergies and schizophrenia simply because the gastric mucosa are affected in the wheat-allergy celiac lesion which is frequently present. Vitamin A is given as 10,000 units three times a day. When vitamin D is used, the dosage range can be from 400 units to 1,250 units three times a day. Both A and D dosages can later be reduced based on individual tolerance and need.

It may be necessary to maintain these high dosages of vitamins two or three months or more in severely allergic patients. After that period of time, the dosage may be maintained at a high level or reduced. This, of course, is a matter of biochemical individuality in each patient. Orthomolecular physicians are specifically trained in the proper dosages of all nutrients.

An initial hair-analysis test, which should be repeated in six months to one year, can serve as a guide to supplementation of necessary minerals. The possibility of toxic levels of lead, mercury, cadmium, or arsenic is also determined by the hair analysis. Knowing how to define the mineral element status of the patient, knowing the clinical signs of deficiencies, imbalances, or toxicities, and defining them is a major part of clinical nutrition. The narrow normal ranges and delicate balances for the major minerals, and especially the trace elements, demand a precise, accurate determination of the patient's mineral-element state. Numerous studies have demonstrated the usefulness of hair as a recording medium of intake and retention of mineral elements. Both essential and toxic elements have been clinically monitored using this method and have clearly indicated reliable correlations between hair elemental values and clinical manifestations of mineral excesses and deficiencies.

Mineral supplements, such as zinc, magnesium, and manganese, are best when provided in chelated form. Chelation means that the mineral is bonded to a protein molecule, giving better absorption and utilization of the mineral. Potassium can be provided as potassium-gluconate tablets. Also, a sodium supplement is sometimes needed, and ordinary sea salt is the best source. When high dosages of B_6 and C are used, it is sometimes advisable to supplement extra sodium and potassium. Calcium is also needed when there is a relatively large amount of vitamin C used. The hair analysis will indicate the need for these and other minerals. It is important to check the hair test against serum calcium, magnesium, zinc, and chromium, which give a picture of the immediate state of affairs. Sometimes high calcium in the hair is caused by a metabolic problem of excessive calcium deposit in the hair in the face of a serum calcium deficiency.

Sometimes there are substances in the vitamin-mineral supplements to which some people are very sensitive. Some tablets will contain cornstarch as a filler; others may have sugar or food colorings in them. Fortunately, some manufacturers are aware of the allergic possibilities of such substances and consequently make their products without these ingredients. In order to avoid any possible misunderstanding or trouble when beginning on a supplement program, one should always be aware of all the ingredients in each supplement. If this is not taken into consideration, complications may arise. If someone is sensitive to hydrocarbons, for example, any supplements that contain coloring may evoke a serious allergic reaction. In such a case, the supplement would do the patient more harm than good. In milk-sensitive people, supplements that contain lactose (milk sugar) must be avoided. If there is any doubt about the supplement, it is advisable to write the manufacturer and inquire about the product.

There are many cases that are not suitable for home diagnosis and treatment of supernutrition. No one knows who these are until testing has been done. A person, for example, may have a B_{12} deficiency, which requires intramuscular injections of B_{12}. This would not be known unless testing was done. The same thing may be true of folic acid. The mineral content of the hair is not known unless a hair analysis is made, and the same is true for the amino-acid content. Toxic minerals such as lead, mercury, or excessive copper may be present and not discovered until testing is done. With toxic metal problems, it is often vital to discover the source of the contamination. There have been patients whose water supply was badly contaminated; there was another case in which the eating of a large amount of tuna created mercury poisoning in the patient; the heavy consumption of tobacco sometimes creates a toxic level of cadmium. I recall one woman whose hair coloring mixture contained lead; she was absorbing it through her scalp, and a severe case of lead poisoning developed in her over the years. These problems and many similar ones will usually not be recognized except by a trained clinician. I must emphasize that you test before you treat, and if you use supplements, know exactly what you are doing, or go to a trained orthomolecular physician who has had thousands of cases that have given him priceless insights into the proper treatment of biochemical deficiencies.

The correct balancing of vitamins, minerals, amino acids, and trace elements is essential in the successful treatment of degenerative disease. But treatment procedures do not stop with these tools. New discoveries about the biochemical functioning of proteolytic enzymes and amino acids, and their use in the treatment of disease, have given orthomolecular physicians a better grasp of the fundamental principle that all nutrients always work best when used together as a team. Therefore, let us turn our attention to some very important players on the team of nutrients necessary for optimum health.

Chapter 6

Proteolytic-Enzyme and Amino-Acid Therapy in Degenerative Disease

Since the 1920s, medical practitioners have been recording individual maladaptive reactions to foods and chemicals observed as emerging during controlled systematic test exposures. As we have seen, these reactions are especially acute after a four-to-six-day period of avoidance of incriminated substances. These reactions have been varyingly characterized as allergic, hypersensitive, and maladaptive or as enzymatic-deficiency reactions. Substances evoking these reactions are far more numerous than the proteins conventionally associated with allergic reactions and include all food categories and chemicals, especially those most frequently contacted. The types of reactions evoked are as varied as the many tissues and organ systems of the human body; therefore, mental as well as physical symptoms can occur.

The pancreas is the first endocrine organ to be influenced by contact with ingested foods and chemicals. It has the monumental task of making useful metabolic products from the ingested substances and also buffering against reactions to any of these substances. An overstimulated pancreas follows the same general law that other overstimulated tissues and organ systems follow: overstimulation eventually leads to inhibition of function. It is well documented that addiction to alcohol (which, of course, overstimulates the pancreas) leads to pancreatic insufficiency. What has been little appreciated is that all addictions, whether they are to foods of any kind, chemicals, tobacco, or alcohol, lead to pancreatic insufficiency of varying degrees. Most affected in pancreatic insufficiency is the bicarbonate production, followed by the organ's enzyme production, and least of all its insulin production.

To understand the significance of pancreatic insufficiency, we need to examine the basic physiology of the pancreas's function. One of its most important systemic functions is to supply proteolytic enzymes (enzymes from the pancreas that aid in the digestion of proteins to amino acids), which act as regulatory mechanisms over inflammatory reactions in the body. Among the several substances in the human body capable of evoking inflammatory reactions are the tissue hormones known as kinins. Kinin reactions are usually the most frequent, the most severe, and the most painful. These hormones are evoked by inflammatory substances (food, chemicals, and so on) to which a person may be allergic. Consequently, symptoms of all kinds are caused by the production of kinin inflammation in specific tissues or organs (including the brain) responding to contact with specific allergy-evoking substances. Proteolytic enzymes have a regulatory and inflammation-resolving control over kinin-mediated inflammation and are capable of actually blocking the rise in kinins. Thus, these substances are powerful enough to prevent the kinin-mediated reaction from occurring. The liver produces the proteolytic enzyme orgotein (superoxide dismutase), which is important in the control of inflammation. The blood contains the proteolytic enzyme fibrinolysin. Heparin is a widespread tissue metabolite, which has powerful anti-inflammatory value.

The consequence of an insufficiency of pancreatic proteolytic enzymes is poor digestion of proteins to amino acids. Proteolytic enzymes are built from amino acids, and if amino acids are deficient, these inflammation-resolving and inflammation-blocking enzymes will also be deficient. More specifically, if amino acids are deficient, they will fail to activate the duodenal and jejunal mucosa to produce cholecystokinin-pancreazyme, which, in turn, evokes proteolytic-enzyme secretions from the pancreas. However, with an amino-acid deficiency, there is more than just a reduced enzyme production from the pancreas. Hormones and antibodies performing their vital functions are reduced in quality and quantity. Excessive demand for vitamins, minerals, and trace elements, especially B_6 and its helpers zinc and magnesium, is also established. This demand sets up a chain of deficiencies, which usually results in a further weakening of pancreatic function, infectious invasion due to unhealthy tissues, and low immunological defenses. But what is most important to understand here is the fact that poor digestion of proteins to amino acids occurs as a consequence of insufficient pancreatic proteolytic enzymes. As a result, unusable inflammation-evoking protein molecules are absorbed through the intestinal mucosa and circulated in the blood, reaching tissues in partially digested form. As partially digested protein molecules (peptides), they are treated as invaders in the body and establish kinin-mediated inflammation in specific organ or tissue targets. This fact becomes of special import when we realize that there is test information justifying the conclusion that two-thirds of all maladaptive reactions to substances to which a patient may be allergic are kinin-mediated inflammatory reactions (nonimmunologic) or other similar inflammatory reactions. The other one-third is antibody histamine-mediated inflammations (immunologic). Edema or tissue swelling, common to both histamine and kinin inflammatory reactions, makes these inflammatory experiences clinically indistinguishable. However, kinin inflammations are more likely to be painful than histamine inflammatory reactions since kinins evoke pain when in contact with nerve endings.

Gastric digestion occurs in an acid medium (pH of 1.8 to 3, with best function occurring at a pH of 1.8 to 2), while the small intestine functions in an alkaline medium of pH 6.8 and higher, and best at a pH of 8 to 9. The pancreas produces bicarbonate, and the fluids coming from the pancreas normally have a pH of 8. It is significant to note that proteolytic enzymes from the pancreas function in a neutral to alkaline medium, and function best in a pH medium of 8 to 9. These enzymes are destroyed in an acid medium. The consequences of insufficient pancreatic bicarbonate (alkaline medium for the enzymes) are:

- acute metabolic acidosis after meals, since the pancreatic bicarbonate has not neutralized the acid from the stomach as it empties into the duodenum
- inactivation of and/or destruction of proteolytic enzymes from the pancreas
- injury to the small intestine's mucosa

In order to avoid metabolic acidosis, bicarbonate is often prescribed with proteolytic enzymes, since the latter cannot function without the former.

A growing number of psychiatrists, who have demonstrated maladaptive reactions to foods and various chemicals to be common in different forms of degenerative disease, are finding that, more often than not, these maladaptive reactions, whether manifested in mental and/or physical symptoms, reveal the presence of pancreatic insufficiency ranging from mild to severe and from reversible to irreversible. These psychiatrists maintain that, since pancreatic proteolytic enzymes (chymotrypsin and carboxypeptidase) are anti-kinin or anti-inflammatory agents, they can in effect be characterized as nature's tranquilizers. That is, nature established that the pancreas has the essential job of providing enzymes that control inflammation, whether due to a cut, a bruise, or a food or chemical allergic reaction in any tissue or organ of the body. Nature has also arranged it so that the pancreatic proteolytic enzymes have no observable feedback mechanism or disease-producing side effects.

In contrast to the "no harm" principle of proteolytic enzymes, the major tranquilizers (phenothiazine), antidepressants (impiramine hydrochloride), and lithium, which many doctors have used in the past few decades to inhibit kinin reactions, have the major disadvantages of frequently producing chronic diseases such as parkinsonism and tardive dyskinesia, as well as a four- to fivefold increase in the incidence of overt clinical diabetes.[32] Moreover, while these drugs do indeed lower kinin inflammation, they do not alter the basic disease process, which continues and may even worsen.

On the other hand, nature's proteolytic enzyme therapy (which effectively controls kinin inflammation without producing clinical side effects), coupled with a proper rotation diet, optimum nutrient intake specifically designed for individual deficiencies, and the elimination of any incriminating food or chemical to which a person has a maladaptive reaction, actually slows down the disease process and can, at times, even reverse physical or mental degeneration.

This is not to say that, since we now have anti-inflammatory enzymes, it no longer matters what a person eats, smokes, or drinks or what her basic nutritional state is. It matters very much! A person cannot be nutritionally deficient, toxic, infected, or addicted to any food or chemical without suffering the consequences of progression of the disease process into a chronic degenerative illness of some type. Providing amino acids, pancreatic proteolytic enzymes, and bicarbonate simply provides physiological supplements in a stress-failing organism. But for reasonably successful treatment, it cannot be overemphasized that all the other dynamics of the human organism must be honored; for example, reduced physiological and psychological stresses, no addictions to any food or chemical (including tobacco and alcohol), optimum nutrition, optimum exercise, optimum rest, and optimum immunological defense against opportunist microbes. As we have already learned previously, symptom-evoking foods, chemicals, and inhalants need to be identified and avoided and thereafter spaced with a frequency below what will occasion symptom production.

In short, pancreatic proteolytic-enzyme therapy is to be viewed as one useful tool among many within the dynamics of orthomolecular-ecological medicine rather than as a patch on inflammations, as has been the practice with chemical tranquilizers, antidepressants, sedatives, and hypnotics.

Brief summaries of three case histories (given in detail in the appendix) demonstrate the dramatic effects of this treatment.

A twenty-six-year-old woman diagnosed as suffering from catatonic schizophrenia showed symptoms of sweating hands, followed by tension progressing to catatonia after a test meal of cheddar cheese. When the test was repeated after two administrations of 1,670 milligrams of concentrated pancreatic enzymes, followed by a quarter-teaspoon of a mixture of sodium bicarbonate and potassium bicarbonate, there was no tension or catatonia and only minor sweating of the hands.

A twenty-seven-year-old woman suffering from chronic schizo-affective reaction displayed a severe diabetic reaction (elevated blood sugar), tension, trembling, irritability, and anger one hour after a test meal of raisins. Repetition of the test, with enzymes administered as in the first case, resulted in no symptoms; blood sugar was normal. Testing with apples gave a similar result.

A twenty-three-year-old schizophrenic man who reacted severely to contact with exhaust fumes, perfumes, and other airborne substances showed only minor improvement when tested for these substances after various enzymes were administered; however, after combining amino acids with the proteolytic enzymes, testing left him free of all but minor physical symptoms—a brief nasal stuffiness at the beginning of the test.

It is unwise to use only proteolytic-enzyme and amino-acid therapy for schizophrenia or other chronic degenerative diseases in the expectation of a miraculous cure. Other nutrient deficiencies, metabolic errors, infections, physical stresses, and emotional stresses must all be kept in mind when attempting to treat severe degenerative diseases. To achieve a dynamic homeostasis equilibrium, all isolatable factors should be treated appropriately and simultaneously. However, it seems apparent that proteolytic-enzyme and amino-acid supplementation will play an important role in the treatment of many chronic degenerative diseases, including the major mental conditions such as schizophrenia, manic-depressive reactions, psychotic depression, and autism. Although I have concentrated here on schizophrenia, it should be understood that it is but one of the chronic degenerative diseases and has characteristics in common with several other chronic degenerative conditions, particularly diabetes mellitus and hypoglycemia. These will be discussed in detail in chapter 10.

Chapter 7

The Healing Powers of Vitamin C

In treating infections of all kinds and their associated symptoms, physicians make wide use of antibiotics. A few years ago when the population was two hundred million, we Americans consumed 4,037,000 pounds of penicillin in one year. There is no doubt that penicillin has saved many lives and has considerably reduced the amount of human suffering in our country. The trouble with all this is that when doctors think entirely in terms of immediate symptomatic relief of specific infections via the use of a broad range of different antibiotics, they ignore the underlying nutritional deficiencies associated with the disease process. Thus, they are closing their eyes to the opportunities to make people's nutritionally supported, immunological defense systems more resistant to future infectious invasion. As a result of this current medical practice, the most fundamental weapons available in the battle against infectious disease are those most ignored by modern medicine: nutrients. This is a gross error since, as I hope I have already demonstrated, the nutritional microenvironment of our body cells is the most crucially important factor involved in maintaining health, and deficiencies in this environment constitute a major cause of disease. More specifically, acute nutritional deficiencies can actually produce a fertile medium for opportunist, infectious organisms to flourish.

Roger J. Williams, Ph.D., past president of the American Chemistry Society, put it succinctly when he said, "If our body cells are ailing, as they must be in disease, then chances are excellent that it is because they are being inadequately provisioned. The list of things that these cells may need includes not only all amino acids and all the minerals, plus trace elements, but about fifteen vitamins and probably many other coenzymes, nutrilites, and metabolites."[33] And as Williams maintains, "Drugs at best are only a palliative form of treatment. . . . The basic fault of these weapons [drugs] is that they have no known connection with the disease process itself. . . . These drugs are wholly unlike nature's weapons [nutrients]. . . . They tend to mask the difficulty, not eliminate it. They contaminate the internal environment, create dependence on the part of the patient, and often complicate the physician's job by erasing valuable clues as to the real source of the trouble."[34] Statistics tell us that as much as 5 percent of all hospital admissions—one and a half million—are now the result of adverse reactions to legally acquired prescription drugs. Once a patient is in the hospital, his chances of acquiring drug-induced sickness more than doubles. This means that over three and a half million people experience drug-induced internal contamination and dependence.

In light of these facts, many physicians are beginning to insist that the primary reliance in the battle against infectious disease—all forms of disease, for that matter—should always be on weapons that are most similar to nature's own biological weapons. With this thought in mind, Linus Pauling coined the term *orthomolecular medicine.* Simply stated: treatment of a disease is a matter of "varying the concentration of substances [i.e., right molecules such as vitamins, minerals, trace elements, hormones, amino acids, enzymes] normally present in the human body."[35] In other words, orthomolecular medicine aims at the achievement and preservation of optimum health and the prevention and treatment of disease by regulating the concentration of chemical molecules normally present in the human body. One of these molecules important in the treatment of infectious disease is vitamin C. To appreciate why an optimum daily intake of this nutrient is so essential in the battle against infectious disease and to well-being in general, we must first remember that we have a genetic defect that prevents us from making our own supply of vitamin C inside our bodies. This is not true for most other animals. They manufacture ascorbic acid—vitamin C—either in their kidneys or in their livers, and thus do not need an external source for this necessary nutrient. The mammals that have been clinically examined in this respect range from a mouse, weighing less than one ounce, to a goat, weighing around 75 pounds, and the amounts of vitamin C manufactured by these two different mammals are approximately proportionate to their body weights. The mouse, for example, is reported to make the equivalent of 19 grams per day, calculated on the basis of 70 killigrams body weight, and the goat 13 grams per day, measured on the same basis. These normal daily levels increase dramatically when the animal is placed under a stress situation, such as an infectious flare-up. Our experience is that nature's workings are in the main balanced, so it would seem safe to assume that it is unlikely that these animals would synthesize more ascorbic acid than needed for optimum health. But the controversial question now arises of precisely what amounts of this particular vitamin are needed to put a person, who does not manufacture vitamin C, in the best of health and give him the greatest immunological protection against infectious diseases of all kinds.

In order to answer this, we must first understand the concept of Recommended Dietary Allowance (RDA) as formulated by the Food and Nutrition Board of the National Academy of Sciences, National Research Council. Most laypeople interpret RDA for any particular nutrient—in this case, vitamin C—as being that specific dosage that leads to the best of health for all people. That is, if I take the RDA of vitamin C every day of my life, I will more than likely achieve the best of health that can possibly be gained by the intake of this nutrient. This interpretation is quite false. The truth of the matter is that the RDA is only the estimated amount that, for most people, will prevent scurvy or death caused by overt vitamin deficiency. It does not take into account biochemical individuality or individual levels of nutrients needed for optimum health. This point is very important and should be understood thoroughly. Dr. Harper, former chairman of the Committee on Recommended Daily Allowances of the Food and Nutrition Board, clearly stated that the RDAs "are not recommendations for the ideal diet." "They were adopted," continued Dr. Hegstedt, another nutritionist, "to avoid any implication of finality or optimal requirements."[36] In short, the board's recommendations were adopted so as to indicate to the general American public those amounts of vitamin C needed in order to avoid scurvy. The same is true, of course, for all the other nutrients and their deficiency-related diseases.

The problem with the board's recommendations is that the medical profession took hold of them and created a misconception now generally accepted by many physicians. This misconception is based on the following reasoning: lack of ascorbic acid causes scurvy. If there are no signs or symptoms of scurvy, we must assume that there is no deficiency whatever of ascorbic acid. Therefore, there is no need to take supplements of this vitamin. The first sentence of this three-part deduction is a medical fact. However, the problem arises with the false assumption that since there are no symptoms of scurvy, there is absolutely no need for any additional intake of vitamin C. You see, scurvy is not just a symptom of lack, but a final collapse, a death syndrome manifesting itself in a total breakdown and disintegration of our biochemical being. But there is a very large gray area (i.e., colds, infections, flu, degenerative disease) existing between the total blackness of scurvy and death and the pure white of optimum health and resistance to disease. It is precisely in this gray area that we must answer the important question: What intake of vitamin C is needed in order to achieve optimum health and resistance to disease rather than barely avoid developing scurvy? No longer can we be satisfied with the misconception that if we do not have scurvy, we do not need any additional amounts of vitamin C in order to achieve the optimum health possible for our particular biochemical being. And no longer can we be satisfied with the uninformed opinion that the RDA alone will guarantee our optimum health. At this point, what we can be guaranteed is that if we do take the RDA of vitamin C, we will very likely not develop scurvy. The question still remains, however: What if a person takes greater amounts of vitamin C than the RDA? Will these greater concentrations of this particular nutrient increase her resistance to infectious and/or degenerative disease and thereby give her better health than if she had not taken them?

According to Linus Pauling, "There is overwhelming clinical evidence that an increased intake of vitamin C, that is, several times the RDA of 45 milligrams per day for an adult, provides significant protection against the common cold."[37] Several double-blind, scientific studies conducted between 1942 and 1975 all confirm Pauling's thinking that an increased intake of ascorbic acid (and other nutrients, of course) strengthens a person's natural protective mechanisms of the body and thus decreases both the number of colds and severity of individual colds. The results of these double-blind studies are shown in the following chart.[38]

Study	*Reduction in Illness*
Cowan, Diehl, Baker: Minnesota, 1942	31%
Ritzel: Switzerland, 1961	63%
Anderson, Reid, Beaton: Canada, 1973	32%
Coulehan, Reisinger, Rogers, Bradley: Arizona, 1974	30%
Charleston, Clegg: Scotland, 1972	58%
Sabiston, Radonski: Canada, 1974	68%
Anderson, Beaton, Corey, Spero: Canada, 1975	25%
Average reduction in illness due to an increased intake of vitamin C	44%

The amounts of ascorbic acid taken in these preceding double-blind studies varied from 200 milligrams to 2,000 milligrams (2 grams). These positive results were achieved because of the functions that vitamin C performs in the body. Therefore, let us examine these functions.

Probably the most important and potent defense mechanism that the body has is the total destruction of invading opportunist and infectious microorganisms by the leukocytes or white blood cells of the blood. This process is called phagocytosis. It was clinically established as long as thirty years ago that vitamin C is one of the most important ingredients for the proper and effective phagocytic activity of leukocytes. Indeed, leukocytes can only maintain their phagocytic activity against infectious microorganisms, engulfing them and destroying them, if the leukocytes contain optimum levels of vitamin C; unless the white blood cells are totally saturated with ascorbic acid, they are like soldiers without bullets. The white blood cells have the ability to ingest the bacterial microorganisms, and when they do, they simultaneously produce hydrogen peroxide. This chemical must then combine with vitamin C to produce a substance that is lethal to almost all known bacteria. If the proper levels of vitamin C are not present at a biochemical war site, the white blood cells' battle against the microorganisms will be lost. Drs. Hume and Weyers, in Scotland, reported in 1973 that an ordinary diet usually does not contain adequate amounts of vitamin C needed for proper phagocytic action of the white blood cells during the stress situation of a cold.[39] Even an intake of 250 milligrams a day is not enough to maintain phagocytically effective amounts. Normally, however, an intake of 1 to 15 grams daily during an infectious stress situation like a cold is enough of a concentration to enable this natural mechanism of protection against bacterial disease to operate. But even these large amounts are sometimes not enough, depending on the specific infectious microorganisms involved.

Many scientists, physicians, and nutritionists have reported that vitamin C in large dosages inactivates all forms of viruses in vitro. Technically speaking, Murata and Kitagawa believe that this inactivation results from the splitting of the nucleic acid of the virus by free radicals formed during the oxidation of vitamin C.[40] Viruses of poliomyelitis, vaccina, hoof and mouth, rabies, hepatitis, pneumonia, measles, chickenpox, mononucleosis, encephalitis, and others have all been destroyed in experiments using optimum dosages of ascorbic acid. When attempting to treat any of the preceding infections with vitamin C, individual optimum dosages of the nutrient are best determined by adopting the principle of "bowel-tolerance level." Robert F. Cathcart, M.D., explains his concept in the following way:

> About seven years ago, I began to hear rumors about Dr. Pauling saying something about vitamin C and the common cold. I had been a person who had suffered all my life with hay fever, having had injections since the age of nine. I was also one of those persons who had colds all the time. So I started taking vitamin C and found that I could give up my injections for hay fever, and also that my colds were under control. But then I went on and discovered something very interesting: I was able to take an amount of vitamin C when I was ill with a cold that I couldn't possibly tolerate when I was well. We elaborated on that a little bit and started experimenting with patients. After clinical testing, we came up with what I call bowel-tolerance concept in determining the dose of vitamin C that should be given patients. . . . Bowel-tolerance levels of vitamin C means you let the body take as much vitamin C as it needs until diarrhea occurs. Once you get diarrhea, you cut back a couple or more grams until the diarrhea goes away. This practice lets the body use that amount of vitamin C proportional to the amount of toxin that is around. . . . The astonishing thing about bowel-tolerance levels of vitamin C is that the same person—who when well gets diarrhea on say 12 grams—with a moderate cold can take 30 to 60 grams without diarrhea; with a bad cold or flu can take 100 to 150 grams; and with viral diseases such as mononucleosis or viral pneumonia can take in excess of 200 grams a day without producing diarrhea. In some cases, the body evidently needs that much, albeit for only a short time. . . . Essentially, the sicker you are, the more you can take, and taking enough—and that is important—seems to detoxify you. You get well quickly! As you do, you will find that you can tolerate less and less ascorbic acid until you go back to normal when you are well. Remember, everyone else has been talking about a fixed dose of vitamin C. Those studies go from 2 to maybe 4 grams a day, and they sometimes see little chemical or statistical effect. That doesn't surprise me. If you have a

> 100-gram flu bug—it's my custom to put a number before the name of the disease to represent the amount of vitamin C that the patient can consume the first couple of days of the disease without diarrhea—and thus take roughly 100 grams of vitamin C, you will quickly eliminate 90 percent of the symptoms of the disease. But if you treat a 100-gram bowel-tolerance-level flu bug with 2 or even 20 grams a day, you will not see much happen.[41]

Figure 7.1 represents Dr. Cathcart's clinical finding concerning average minimum dosages of vitamin C per twenty-four hours needed to neutralize acute symptoms of disease.

Note that the amount of vitamin C necessary to produce diarrhea increases more or less proportionately to the toxicity of the disease. Bowel-tolerance levels of vitamin C are obviously greater for pneumonia than they are for a severe cold. Also, these levels increase somewhat according to the degree of other stress-related factors: al-

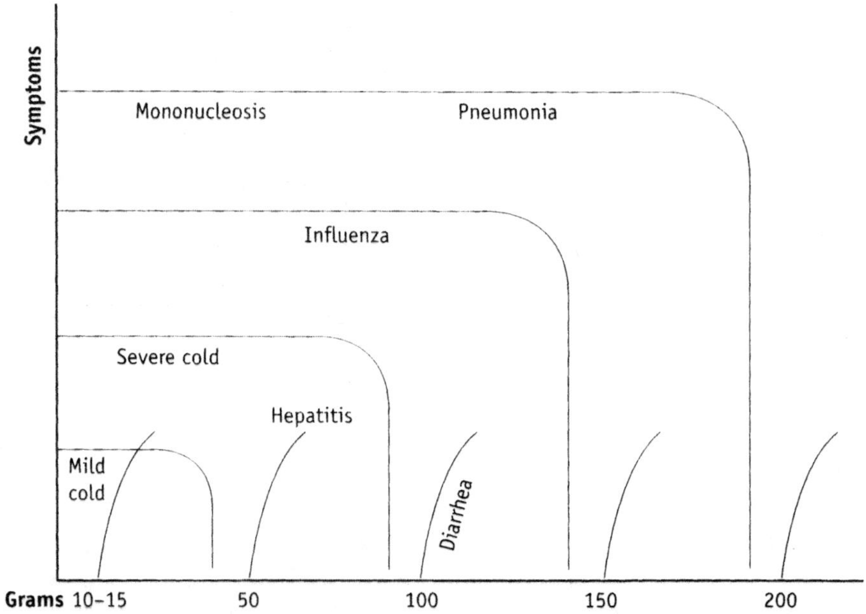

FIGURE 7.1. *Dr. Cathcart's minimum dose of vitamin C per twenty-four hours to neutralize acute symptoms of disease.*

lergy, heat, cold, anxiety, drinking, cancer, injury, surgery, psychosis, arthritis, and so on. It is important to understand that 80 percent of people tolerate 0.5 to 10 grams of ascorbic acid when well; most of the remainder get diarrhea somewhere in these levels. However, when those who tolerate it poorly are sick, their tolerance approaches the levels of the other 80 percent.

Acute symptoms are affected very little until 90 percent of the bowel tolerance is reached. The symptoms drop off suddenly. This is the reason the symptom curve is drawn flat at first and then suddenly drops (see Figure 7.1). Also, symptoms may not clear completely in severe cases. In these cases, intravenous or intramuscular injections will abolish all symptoms. This clinical form of treatment should be reserved for very toxic illnesses or for those who do not tolerate ascorbic acid well by mouth. Frederick R. Klenner, M.D., has had over thirty years of clinical work with vitamin C and explains precisely how shots should be given:

> Effecting a cure when a virus is the offending agent, and many times bringing about this change in the short space of twenty-four hours, is a rewarding moment in medicine. Vitamin C treatment must be intensive to be successful. Use veins when practical, otherwise give vitamin C intramuscularly. Never give less than 350 milligrams per kilogram body weight. This must be repeated every hour for up to twelve times, depending upon clinical improvement, then every two to four hours until the patient has recovered. Ice cubes held to the gluteal muscle before and after injection will reduce or eliminate pain and induration. When treatment continues for several days, the person can be placed on an ice cap between injections. When employing vitamin C intravenously, it is best to use sodium ascorbate and the solution free of all additives except sodium bisulfite. The dose of vitamin C using a syringe should range between 350 milligrams and 400 milligrams per kilogram body weight. In older patients, or when very high doses are required, the vitamin can be added to 5 percent dextrose in water, in saline solution, or in Ringer's solution. The concentration should be approximately 1 gram to 18 cc fluid. Bottle injections will need

> 1 gram calcium gluconate one to two times each day to replace calcium ions removed by the high intravenous schedule. One quart of milk daily will suffice when using the vitamin intramuscularly. Or in the place of milk one can substitute calcium-gluconate tablets. Supplemental vitamin C is always given by mouth. As a guide in determining the amount and frequency of injection, we recommend our silver nitrate-urine test. This is done by placing ten drops of 5 percent silver nitrate in a Wasserman tube and adding ten drops of urine. A color pattern will develop showing white, beige, smoke gray, or one that looks like fine-grain charcoal. Charcoal is the color needed, and the test is performed at least every four hours. The test itself is read in one minute. . . . The killing power of vitamin C is not limited. When proper amounts are used it will destroy virus organisms. . . . By 1950, we learned that we could kill the measles virus in twenty-four hours by giving intramuscular injections in a dose range of 350 milligrams per kilogram body weight every two hours. We also found that we could dry up chickenpox in the same time, but more dramatic results were obtained by giving 400 milligrams per kilogram body intravenously. In conclusion, the killing power of ascorbic acid on virus bodies has been demonstrated by me in hundreds of cases, many of which were treated in our hospital with nothing but vitamin C.[42]

When a person has been taking large doses of vitamin C for a few weeks or longer, the amount of this nutrient in his blood is such that if he suddenly stops taking high dosages of it, blood levels of ascorbic acid will be rapidly converted into other substances, and the concentration of vitamin C in the blood will become abnormally low. This "rebound effect," as Dr. Pauling calls it, will, in turn, decrease one's resistance to further infectious flare-up.[43] Accordingly, it is wise for one who has been on a large dosage of vitamin C to decrease the intake gradually over a week or two, rather than suddenly. When decreasing vitamin C dosages, bowel-tolerance levels should be maintained until you are completely well. Then continue to take your daily prophylactic dose of the nutrient.

In order for us really to appreciate the healing powers of vitamin C, we should look briefly at some firsthand reports of clinical cases in which this nutrient was given in large dosages. Dr. Cathcart gives us some excellent examples of these clinical situations in which pneumonia, mononucleosis, and hepatitis—illnesses so severe that traditional medical techniques, such as the use of antibiotics, can often take as long as a month or more to rehabilitate the patient—are effectively treated with vitamin C in less than a week. Of course, the patients must continue to take their individually determined bowel-tolerance levels of vitamin C for some time or until they are completely well. But, basically, their severe symptoms disappear three to five days after taking vitamin C in large dosages, and they are able to continue their daily living patterns.

Pneumonia

Let me give you a typical case. A twenty-eight-year-old woman developed viral pneumonia. As far as I could tell, she did not respond to antibiotics, and she never did "culture" any place. When she presented herself, she was very ill with a high temperature, the right upper lobe infiltrated with the pneumonia process, and difficulty breathing. So we hooked her up to intravenous ascorbic acid, about 1 gram per 18 cc, and ran it in just as fast as we could. I gave her about 55 grams by vein and the remainder orally; about 215 grams went into her between eleven o'clock in the morning and nine o'clock that night, at which time the pneumonia went into crisis. She drenched three sets of bed clothing that night. The next morning she was feeling much better. We did the same thing the next day. She returned to work less than a week after I saw her. We have daily X rays that demonstrate the rapid dissolution of the pneumonia process.

At that time, I treated two other people in town who had the same thing and got similar results. Three other patients in town went to other physicians and were hospitalized for about two weeks and weren't much better when they came out.

Mononucleosis

The first patient that I ran into with mononucleosis was a junior high school librarian who was about twenty-two and weighed about 100 pounds wringing wet. She came in with a severe case of mononucleosis. I told her about the bowel-tolerance idea and explained to her how to do this self-titration. I saw her three or four days later; she was almost completely well. The typical patient who gets mononucleosis is exactly the one who does the best on vitamin C: older teenagers or young adults are just fantastic vitamin C takers. They can understand the bowel-tolerance idea, have iron stomachs, and couldn't care less about slight gas and diarrhea when they have this horrible disease. In fact, the sicker the patient is the better he does because the relief of symptoms is so dramatic that he doesn't need any arguments to convince him to continue treatment. What usually happens is that in three to five days the symptoms are 90 percent relieved. Then the patient must get the message loud and clear: If he stops the vitamin C too soon, he will get sick all over again.

Hepatitis

The other disease that is very specific is infectious hepatitis. It's a cinch for vitamin C. The difference between the course of the disease with and without vitamin C is quite obvious if only because hepatitis is a disease that we can put numbers on. There are various enzyme systems that we can follow to show the course of the disease. Infectious hepatitis can be mild where the patient is just a little yellow and maybe a bit tender in the abdomen, but not very sick. But the patients I'm talking about—twenty of them, at least—were profoundly ill with hepatitis, and again we were able to detoxify them in three to five days. In two or three days the urine returned to normal color; in three to four days patients felt essentially well; and it generally took six days for the jaundice to clear.

Hepatitis is a very serious problem, especially following blood transfusions. The whole system of gathering blood in this country is undergoing a revision because people who sell their blood have a high incidence of hepatitis. One of the most important clinical observations concerning prevention of hepatitis after transfusions was made by two Japanese physicians. Drs. Murata and Morishige discovered that an intake of more than 2 grams a day of vitamin C protects surgical patients who receive blood transfusions against serum hepatitis. There was about a 7 percent hepatitis level in their hospital. Then over 1,100 patients in the hospital were given 2 grams of vitamin C daily. The physicians in charge expected at least 70 of the 1,100 to develop hepatitis, but not a single patient developed the viral disease after having taken the vitamin C.[44]

As previously discussed, infections are a very important link in the chain of events that makes up the biochemical disease process. Infections weaken the biochemical system enough to create more serious nutritional deficiencies and thus more severe allergic sensitivity. The infections the patient is harboring, therefore, should always be a part of the differential diagnosis of possible causes of symptoms, both physical and mental. Vitamin C is obviously only one orthomolecular method by which infectious invasion can be controlled. An optimum supply of all the other nutrients is needed as well: amino acids, minerals, and other vitamins. Vitamin B_6 and pantothenic acid, for example, are very important in dealing with the stress of infectious invasion. Vitamin C, of course, is one very powerful weapon we can use in the battle against infectious disease. And when we can better control infections, we simultaneously begin to control the further development of allergic sensitivities.

One point that needs to be discussed in detail before we finish our chapter on vitamin C is the relationship existing between smoking, addiction, and this all-important nutrient. Tobacco is close to being a universal allergen for the human race. Its yearly sales are in the millions of dollars. It is not well known, however, that tobacco smoke contains toxic levels of many gaseous pollutants: carbon monoxide, hydrocyanic acid, nitric oxide, sulfur dioxide, and acetonitrile. The levels of concentration of these pollutants are much higher than might be expected. In addition, the smoke contains finely dispersed carcinogenic tars, poisons such as nicotine, radioactive dust, and other harmful ingredients. Due to the concentration of all these pollutants, the first cigarette smoked causes symptoms such as nausea, dizziness, weakness, and sometimes other, more severe symptoms. These symptoms are due to an allergic reaction to one or all of the preceding pollutants. As with all addictions, persistent use of tobacco causes these symptoms to become delayed in time and even temporarily and partially relieved by smoking again. This physiological compensation for an allergy is termed addiction.

The end result of a frequently evoked allergy, or an allergic-addictive state, is a disturbed metabolic condition leading to chronic physical, emotional, or mental illness. Allergic reactions or allergic-addictive withdrawal symptoms to tobacco can influence any organ system of the body, including the brain. There is much physical as well as mental misery caused by tobacco allergy-addiction. It is common knowledge that tobacco allergy can affect the eyes, sinuses, throat, lungs, stomach, intestines, and vascular system, but it is not usually appreciated that the brain can also be severely disturbed by tobacco addiction. Provocative allergy testing consisting of chain smoking after a four-day withdrawal period has revealed that a hypersensitive tobacco-allergic person can experience a remarkable range of harmful emotional and mental reactions during testing. These can include mild or severe anxiety, tension, fatigue, weakness, perceptual distortions, delusions, and hallucinations.

Even more interesting is the discovery, through allergy-testing techniques, that the desire to smoke is sometimes evoked as a symptom of an allergic reaction to substances other than tobacco. A patient who had never been able to stop smoking on his own was hospitalized, fasted on well water only for four days, and was then fed meals of single foods. The first two days of the fast, his desire to smoke seemed overpowering. By the fourth day of the fast, only a weak impulse to smoke occasionally occurred, but was easily dismissed. Food testing gave evidence of allergic reactions to four different foods. Two of these foods caused, as a part of the reaction, an insatiable urge to smoke. As a result of the hospital experience, he learned that by abstaining from the allergic foods, he found it easier to stop smoking. What this proves is that it is very important to handle all hypersensitive allergic reactions to foods, chemicals, and/or inhalants together in order to arrive at the most successful treatment of addictions.

There are numerous reports in medical literature that tobacco smoke actually destroys ascorbic acid in the body. For example, as far back as 1952, W. J. McCormick stated:

> In determining the anti-infectious protective dosage of vitamin C there is another factor which is not generally considered. When the vitamin is employed to neutralized toxins of endogenous or exogenous origin, the action is reciprocal in that the vitamin is also neutralized proportionately, leaving less available for physiological needs. To illustrate, the writer has determined by laboratory and clinical tests that the smoking of one cigarette neutralizes in the body approximately 25 milligrams of vitamin C, or the amount in one medium-sized orange. It will thus be seen how difficult it is to meet the bodily requirement of the pack-a-day smoker for even the protective level of vitamin C from dietary sources. It is thus obvious that the steady smoker, who is usually short of his dietary intake as well, requires a much heavier therapeutic dosage of this vitamin than the nonsmoker.[45]

Vitamin C has metabolic values beyond its vitamin value. One of these values is that of detoxification. Taking large doses of the nutrient during the four-day withdrawal period will decrease the withdrawal symptoms as well as the urge to smoke. Usually 20 to 30 grams per twenty-four hours can be tolerated without undue symptoms. The most likely symptom with these large doses is diarrhea. However, it is an inconsequential symptom compared to the value ascorbic acid has in relieving withdrawal symptoms. If diarrhea develops, the ascorbic acid intake should be slightly reduced. Ascorbic acid should be taken during the four-day withdrawal period and then stopped during the food and chemical testing period. Tablets or capsules should be avoided, if possible, since they often contain cornstarch and/or other foods and can thus interfere with food testing. Pure ascorbic-acid powder is preferable. Fine-powdered ascorbic acid is best tolerated by many people. Calcium ascorbate is best tolerated by a few. The minimum should be one teaspoon four times a day; double this if possible and if well tolerated. It is better to divide the dosages into six or eight doses a day. This insures a frequent detoxification of the tobacco withdrawal symptoms. Each teaspoon of ascorbic-acid powder contains approximately 4 grams of vitamin C. These dosages can be tolerated better by some people if mixed with baking soda in the ratio of one-half baking soda to that of ascorbic acid, mixed in water. The ascorbic acid then becomes sodium ascorbate. Vitamin C can also be purchased as sodium ascorbate. Also, in relieving tobacco-withdrawal symptoms, it can be helpful to use 500 milligrams of pyridoxine, six times in twenty-four hours during the days of withdrawal.

Fasting, combined with the use of certain nutrients, causes the urge to smoke to be postponed rather than acted upon. In this fashion, time is allowed for both the physiologically driven, addictive withdrawal state and the overlearned, habitual aspect of the response to subside. The learned, habitual aspect of smoking is easily unlearned if the strong, driving biological addictive urges are handled first. To treat the smoking habit as a purely learned response is like fighting two opponents singlehandedly. That is, while you concentrate on the learned responses, the undealt-with biological urges keep activating the response to smoke. Therefore, handle the biological problem first by the use of fasting and nutrients; then unlearning that learned habit will be much easier.

When an urge to smoke strikes, the patient is to look at a watch and affirm that she will wait five minutes before deciding whether or not to smoke. This five-minute postponement allows the urge to subside. Habitual responses reach their highest peak in three minutes. It is better, still, to be involved during the postponement period in an active practice that has canceling value to the response; jogging, a vigorous walk, eating a nonallergic food, taking more ascorbic acid, or practicing a behavioral drill with smoking-inhibiting response value may all prove to be helpful in this regard.

I want to digress a little from the main thread of my argument here and enlarge on the role of behavioral drills in a successful program of breaking the addiction to smoking. This is one of the most difficult yet most positive steps in promoting health. Behavioral drills or training should begin the day withdrawal of tobacco and allergic foods begins. The following information, while only marginally related to the function of vitamin C, can be very helpful to those of my readers who wish to stop smoking.

1. With your eyes closed and while relaxed, place in mind the urge to smoke. Take a breath and hold that breath until the picture leaves the mind. This creates an inhibition of the imaged response to smoke by producing an oxygen deficit to which the brain is very sensitive. When an oxygen deficiency occurs, it is very difficult for the brain to maintain any image intact; thus, the urge-to-smoke image is lost. Most people can indeed hold their breath long enough to produce this desired oxygen deficit in their brain.
2. Again place in mind the image of the desire to smoke and then immediately conjure up the image of an unpleasant situation, such as smelling a skunk and vomiting all over your cigarettes, your friends, and their cigarettes.
3. Then call to mind a situation in which you usually smoke—such as while having a cup of coffee—but now see an image of yourself not smoking; feel a sense of value and give yourself credit for not smoking. Then immediately think of the most pleasant situation you can imagine, such as a vacation in Hawaii. Or, an alternative to this pleasant

> imagery is to take three deep breaths while imagining not smoking and being complimented for your success. These three deep breaths activate the adaptive correction of not smoking. Relax again and repeat the imagery sequence. Relax all over and progressively relax parts of the body by letting every muscle go limp; think of your right foot, let every muscle go; then think heavy, heavy, heavy, warm, warm, warm, heavy, warm, relaxed, and so on. Progress to other parts of the body with each drill sequence relaxing a separate part of the body. The cues of heavy, warm, and relax are to be at three-second intervals.

Practice these three drills over and over for fifteen to thirty minutes at a time, six to eight times a day, if possible, whenever tempted to smoke. In the pocket where you keep your cigarettes, or preferably in an empty cigarette package in that pocket, place a small card with the question: What is a good reason not to smoke? Each time you feel like reaching for a cigarette, pull out this card and reflect on an answer to the question. Each person should contemplate the answer that fits him best. The answer might be: It drives me crazy; it can cause cancer of the lungs, an allergic cough, or even heart attacks; it can shorten my life span. There are a great many valid answers. Another useful inhibition to an urge to smoke is to have on one wrist a rubber band, which is snapped vigorously, producing pain. This pain can give immediate inhibition to the urge to smoke and should be followed by the above drill when possible.

The more frequently the corrective behavioral practices are engaged in, the faster the corrective learning will occur. During the four days of withdrawal from tobacco and allergic foods, the practices of breath-holding inhibition of smoking, unpleasant associations with smoking, and pleasant associations with not smoking should be part of every maneuver to handle the urge to smoke. When there is an urge to smoke, then walk or jog, take vitamin C, or go and breathe some pure oxygen while contemplating how good it is not to smoke, and thus agree to postpone smoking until the behavioral drill is engaged in. By this time, the urge will have been significantly reduced and reason will again win over the learned habitual response. Continue to practice these drills until the learned habit of smoking no longer automatically asserts itself.

One of the most important functions of vitamin C in the human body is to maintain biochemical normality under the effects of environmental stress. The term *stress* covers a wide variety of different conditions. Stresses can include hazards to which we are exposed by contact, breathing, eating, smoking, infection, and so on.

One group of chemical hazards not normally considered as a source of stress is poisonous metals. These include the mercury in the seafood we eat, the lead in the gas fumes we inhale, and the hazardous industrial pollution to which we are exposed to some degree almost daily.

It is estimated that at least one million children in the United States have some degree of lead poisoning. This toxic metal's damaging effects are found in an even greater degree in the adult population. Major sources of lead poisoning range from such commonly encountered substances as industrial pollution, paint and auto exhaust, to less obvious ones, such as hair color dyes absorbed through the scalp or drinking water. As far back as 1939, a study of 400 workers in a large industrial plant where the exposure to lead hazards was very great demonstrated the beneficial effect vitamin C in small doses had on these men.[46] Though only 100 milligrams of ascorbic acid were given to each worker, the researcher reported the following results: "Most of the men enjoyed normal sleep, lost the irritability and nervousness so common with high calcium treatment of lead poisoning, enjoyed their food more, and no longer had tremors. Also, several cases of leukopenia (low white blood cell count) were cured by the ascorbic acid treatment."[47] The researcher concluded that vitamin C has a detoxifying action on lead in the body.

The same can be said for the effects of vitamin C on mercury. In 1964, Mokranjac and Petrovic studied the effects of mercury chloride in guinea pigs, tested in groups of twenty-five, where ascorbic acid was administered in different ways.[48] First they gave each animal 200 milligrams of vitamin C a day for one week—roughly equivalent to a 14-gram dose in a human being—which was necessary since the guinea pig, like humans, is one of the few animals that does not manufacture its own supply of ascorbic acid in the liver. The researchers then administered a dose of mercury previously determined to be fatal. They continued to give 200 milligrams of vitamin C daily. After twenty days, all the animals were alive, proving that vitamin C had protected them from certain death. If they gave vitamin C before and none after poisoning, nine of the twenty-five died. If they gave a single massive shot of the nutrient after the poisoning, eight of twenty-five died. This study again confirms our conviction that high daily intake of vitamin C will protect one from many of the ills arising from toxic metal poisoning.

Studies indicate that vitamin C is also a powerful detoxifier of organic poisons such as drugs, tetanus, botulism, and snake venom and can even reverse shock caused by certain drugs. In one patient, who had taken 2,640 milligrams of Lotusate (talbutal), the blood pressure was 60/0 when first seen in the emergency room. Twelve grams of sodium ascorbate was administered with a 50-cc syringe. In ten minutes, the blood pressure was recorded at 100/60. Over a hundred additional grams were given intravenously over the following three hours, at which time the patient was awake and feeling better. Patients in shock from toxalbumin, neurotoxin, proteotoxin, muscarine, and formic acid respond equally well to high dosages of ascorbic acid.

The individual biochemical variations in the need for vitamin C are already an established fact. If we desire, in the treatment of infectious and degenerative disease in general and mental illness in particular, to provide the optimum molecular environment or the optimum concentration of substances normally present in the human body, ascorbic acid should certainly be included. There are numerous studies that suggest that the optimum intake of vitamin C for most mentally ill people can range from 10 to 100 and even 1,000 times the RDA. One of these controlled, double-blind studies of ascorbic acid in chronic psychiatric patients was reported in 1963 by G. Milner.[49] There were forty chronically ill male patients, thirty-four of whom had schizophrenia, four had manic-depressive psychosis, and two had general paresis. Twenty of these men, selected at random, received 1 gram of vitamin C a day for three weeks; the rest received placebo treatment. After the three-week period, the patients were checked by the use of psychological tests. The MMPI and the WPRS were used before and after the trial. Milner concluded, "statistically significant improvement in the depressive, manic, and paranoid symptom complexes, together with an improvement in overall personality functioning, was obtained following saturation with ascorbic acid." The researchers of this double-blind study concluded that improvement could be expected in many psychiatric patients with the use of large dosages of ascorbic acid.

Pauling discovered that of a group of 106 schizophrenic patients, 81 of them (76 percent) were deficient in ascorbic acid, as demonstrated by the six-hour excretion in the urine of less than 17 percent of an orally administered dose. Only 27 of 89 (30 percent) of a group of control subjects showed this deficiency. Very serious deficiencies of vitamin C (less than 4 percent excreted in the urine) were shown by 24 (22 percent) of the schizophrenic subjects and by only 1 (1 percent) of the controls. "I have no doubt," writes Pauling, "that many schizophrenics would benefit from an increased intake of ascorbic acid. My estimate is that 4 grams of vitamin C a day, in addition to the conventional treatment, would increase the fraction of acute schizophrenics in whom the disease is permanently controlled by about 25 percent."[50] Our clinical experience with schizophrenics and vitamin C echoes Pauling's views, though the doses we use are much larger.

Before concluding this chapter on vitamin C, we should direct our attention toward one specific criticism of the use of large dosages of the nutrient. This criticism centers on the relationship existing between the formation of kidney stones and the taking of large amounts of ascorbic acid. First of all, we should understand that there are different types of kidney stones. The tendency to form kidney stones of the ordinary type, phosphate stones, is actually lessened by keeping the urine acidic. Vitamin C, of course, can accomplish this very easily and effectively. However, *The Medical Letter* and *Consumer Reports* have written that persons with a tendency to form kidney stones of the urate and cystine types would at all times keep their urine alkaline. These two scientific reports further point out that vitamin C might increase the chances of causing these stones to form because of its tendency to make the urine more acidic. In such rare cases, ascorbic acid should not be eliminated entirely; rather, it should merely be changed in its form. That is, ascorbic acid is in fact alkaline if the sodium ascorbate form of the nutrient is used. This alkaline form of vitamin C is just as effective in treatment as is the acid form; the only difference is that it will make the urine alkaline and materially reduce the chances of kidney stones developing in patients with such a tendency. My clinical use of megadoses of ascorbic acid and sodium ascorbate as well as such use by others I know causes us to agree with the observation of unlikely production of kidney stones as reported by H. L. Newbold, M.D.[51]

Concern has also developed in the orthodox medical community over the possibility of increasing the amount of oxalic acid in the urine as a result of taking large amounts of vitamin C. All of us normally excrete a small amount of a substance called oxalate everyday. However, when large quantities of oxalate are excreted, calcium-oxalate kidney stones can be formed; and it is true that a few people who take large amounts of vitamin C start to produce abnormally high levels of oxalate, which is then excreted by the kidneys. The normal level of oxalate production is around 40 milligrams or less per twenty-four hours. With an increased intake of vitamin C, this can rise very quickly to 300 to 400 milligrams, which is definitely too high. Is this then sufficient reason for stopping our intake of larger doses of vitamin C? The answer to this question is an emphatic *no*. The researchers who did the studies on levels of oxalate and vitamin C intake were not aware of the fact that vitamin B_6 will actually prevent vitamin C-induced oxalate formation.[52]

There was a patient who, when he began taking 8 grams of vi–tamin C daily, discovered that his oxalate level skyrocketed from 40 to 383 milligrams. When he learned of this, he became very depressed because he thought he would have to stop taking the nutrient. He knew from past experiences that vitamin C at bowel-tolerance levels had offered him many advantages. His conflict was immediately resolved upon a physician's recommendation that he take 50 milligrams of vitamin B_6 twice daily along with his 8 grams of vitamin C. After only two weeks of such treatment, his urinary oxalate test dropped to a little less than 57 milligrams. Vitamin B_6 had saved the day. Our patient was also very happy to discover that he could actually take up to 1,500 milligrams of vitamin C daily by itself without suffering an increase in his urinary oxalate-excretion levels.

This case points to two very important nutritional rules. First, we must always keep in mind biochemical individuality when making scientific studies. What is biologically true for one person might not be at all true for another, even if they are of the same age, sex, and general health pattern. Each person is an individual and reacts individually to every event. In the case of our patient, he could tolerate 1,500 milligrams of vitamin C daily without suffering an increase in his urinary oxalate excretion. You, however, might be able to tolerate ten times that amount. It all depends on biochemical individuality. This principle was recognized as far back as thirteen years ago in *The Heinz Handbook of Nutrition:*

> Individual organisms differ in their genetic makeup and differ also in morphologic and physiologic aspects, including their endocrine activity, metabolic efficiency, and nutritional requirements. . . . It is often taken for granted that the human population is made up of individuals who exhibit average physiologic requirements and that a minor proportion of this population is composed of those whose

> requirements may be considered to deviate excessively. Actually there is little justification in nutritional thinking for the concept that a representative prototype of Homo sapiens is one who has average requirements with respect to all essential nutrients and thus exhibits no unusually high or low needs. In light of contemporary genetic and physiologic knowledge and the statistical interpretations thereof, the typical individual is more likely to be one who has average needs with respect to many essential nutrients but who also exhibits some nutritional requirements for a few essential nutrients, which are far from average.[53]

Unfortunately, this statement has not been generally accepted by the medical establishment. However, orthomolecular physicians are making a serious attempt, not only to discover more about the general ranges of human needs but also to determine specifically for individuals what needs they may have that are far from average.

The second rule of nutrition that was reaffirmed by our case study is known as the teamwork principle. Williams was the first scientist to strongly emphasize this rule. Simply stated, it suggests that nutrients never act singly in the body, but always function together as a team. Williams describes his principle in more detail:

> The fourth basic fact in nutrition, which has been sadly neglected by medical science, is that of the essential "teamwork" among nutrients. Because this principle has been neglected, a wholly unscientific concept has been widely accepted with respect to what a nutrient may be expected to do.
>
> The basic error, tacitly accepted, may be expressed as follows. Nutrients—amino acids, minerals, and particularly vitamins—are potential "medicines," and should be tested accordingly, using statistical methods and suitable placebo controls to determine their efficacy in combating diseases. If they prove to be "specifics" for particular diseases, well and good; if not, they must be regarded as medically worthless. . . .
>
> Following this erroneous reasoning, it is concluded that since

> specific individual nutrients are ineffective when tested in this way against specific common ailments, these nutrients are worthless for combating disease. It is easy to conclude also that there should be no substantial concern regarding the intake of these nutrients on the part of the patients.
>
> The joker in the argument is that while no nutrient by itself is an effective remedy for any common disease, the nutrients acting as a team are probably effective in the prevention of a host of diseases. . . .
>
> It must be emphasized that adequate nutrition must involve the complete chain of nutrients. If a diet is missing one link in the nutritional chain, it may be as worthless for supporting life as if it were missing ten links. One nutrient, such as a mineral, amino acid, or vitamin, added as a supplement to a food can bring no favorable effect unless the food contains some of all the other nutrients or unless they are available from the reserves of the person being nourished.[54]

Drugs are chemical substances which, even if given singly, radically alter man's metabolic machinery and many times interfere with normal vitamin, mineral, amino-acid, and enzyme activities in the body. Nutrients, on the other hand, working as a team, act constructively as building blocks for life in general; without them human life could not exist. Life can exist without drugs! Therefore, nutrients are not drugs and really should not be researched one at a time. In the case of our patient who formed calcium-oxalate kidney stones, it would have been wrong to advise him, based on the clinical research concerning the single study of vitamin C and oxalate levels in the urine, never to take an increased amount of ascorbic acid. The supplement of vitamin B_6 immediately stopped this rare occurrence of the formation of calcium-oxalate kidney stones. Therefore, research must in the future take into account all the interactions of the different nutrients before any scientific conclusions are made.

Moreover, we must remember that no one nutrient, vitamin C included, cures anything by itself. While vitamin C does have many positive effects in the battle against infectious and degenerative diseases, it alone, without all the other nutrients being supplied on an individually determined basis, is practically worthless. So remember, nutrients are always team players. Every kind of organism derives its sustenance from food supplies containing teams of nutrients. The teamwork principle has a very long history; it has been in action consistently and universally ever since life began on earth and still governs our biochemical being.

Chapter 8

Understanding the Disease Process

Toximolecular psychiatrists (those who use drugs or synthetic substances not normally found in the human body) may think they are practicing scientific medicine, but they are not. Even though tranquilizers are helpful at times, they are actually little more than superior sedatives. They sometimes manage to control psychiatric symptoms, but the underlying disease process responsible for the symptoms in the first place usually remains unchecked. What is even more disturbing is the fact that patients on drugs often have to pay a high price for their symptomatic relief by running the statistically high risk of becoming permanently incarcerated in their chemical straitjackets. The result of this type of pharmacological incarceration can vary from such severe side effects as silent coronary death, tardive dyskinesia, parkinsonism, and an increase in the possibility of developing clinical diabetes, to a zombielike, miserable life of social incompetence. Dr. Robert Okin, former Commissioner of Mental Health in Massachusetts, said, "Many patients who had been institutionalized for years now find themselves living in low-cost rooming houses, rocking in front of TV sets, and wandering in the streets."

Many patients are readmitted to the hospital over and over again. Most of them add to the ranks of the unemployed; in fact, statistics tell us that very few tranquilized patients pay income taxes throughout the years of their illness. "The development of toximolecular medicine," writes Humphry Osmond, M.D., "rightly considered a revolution in psychiatry, has not solved the main problems facing this specialty. The flight from the mental hospitals has merely transferred the problem from a concentrated area, the hospitals, to a less concentrated one, the community. The whole community has become the mental hospital."[55] Possibly this exodus of tranquilized yet fundamentally sick individuals into the community is why a British study discovered that the number of institutionalized patients discharged during a one-year period who committed a crime for which they appeared in court increased from 6,366 in 1961 to 12,530 in 1974—almost double the amount!

Toximolecular medicine demands only one thing from its patients—that they continue to take their tranquilizers; but this is not enough. Orthomolecular-ecologic medicine, by contrast, makes the more extended but reasonable demand of its patients that they alter their entire lifestyles in order to optimize their chances of ultimate recovery. This is accomplished by adopting the following procedures:

1. optimum dietary nutrition
2. elimination of all allergy-producing substances, chemicals, or foods, as well as all addictions
3. rotation of foods
4. compensation for nutritional deficiencies via the use of nutrient supplements such as vitamins, minerals, trace elements, enzymes, amino acids, and hormones
5. elimination of toxic minerals such as lead, mercury, arsenic, cadmium, and the like
6. elimination of infections via the use of autogenous vaccines and proper levels of specific nutrients

Granted, these procedures demand more of the patient than the mere popping of a tranquilizer into the mouth. However, such comprehensive orthomolecular-ecologic life-restyling therapy gives promise of reducing or eliminating the disease process itself. Such a therapy stands in contrast to the merely palliative treatment of symptoms, which allows the underlying biochemical degenerative process to continue uninterrupted. Abram Hoffer, M.D., Ph.D., has warned that he has seen many hyperactive young children who were placed on symptomatic drug therapy (e.g., Ritalin®), a type of therapy that brings the hyperactive symptoms immediately under control, later degenerate further into adult schizophrenia because the underlying metabolic problems remained untreated.[56]

An in-depth understanding of the degenerative disease process will enlighten the reader as to why this can occur. For now, however, let us concede that the patient wearing the tranquilizer straitjacket is really in a biochemical prison from which he has no healthy escape. We must begin to realize the necessity for concentrating not on the outward symptoms of the disease, and the resulting toximolecular symptomatic treatment, but on the underlying metabolic disease process itself, and the orthomolecular-ecologic treatment methods by which it can be brought under control.

The orthomolecular-ecologic profile applied to degenerative disease reveals dynamic interactions between several organic factors. These are the common denominators of many different degenerative diseases. The different diseases we all know (i.e., schizophrenia, hyperactivity, diabetes, hypoglycemia, and many others) are named according to the specific tissues inflamed, the particular metabolic systems interfered with, the secondary invading opportunist organisms evoked, the behavioral symptoms displayed, or the specific gland which is disordered; however, the underlying disease process, and its related organic factors, is the basic foundation from which all these different reactions are built.

Hans Selye taught us that there is a central factor in all degenerative diseases.[57] He called this factor *stress*, which he maintained fatigues all biochemical metabolic processes. In our clinic, biochemical monitoring reveals that maladaptive reactions, such as the chronic addictive reactions and their counterpart allergic reactions to foods, chemicals, and inhalants, are the central stress building blocks from which many degenerative diseases are constructed.

As we have already demonstrated in our clinical studies, the frequency with which a food is eaten largely determines whether it becomes a stress burden on the metabolic process. However, dietary patterns are obviously not the only stress factor involved in the disease process. The nutritional quality of the food is very important, since every cell in our body needs the forty-plus nutrients previously mentioned in order to sustain and propagate itself in a healthy manner.

Monitoring of blood-sugar levels, insulin production, acid-base balance, and pancreatic bicarbonate and enzyme production before and after test exposures to potentially allergic substances reveals that the pancreas is the first organ to develop inhibited function from these varied stresses; frequently eaten foods usually are the most obvious stress-producing factors. If the frequency of foods eaten is too great, so as to establish allergic-addictive reactions, or if the nutrient quality is inferior, so as to establish deficiencies in vitamins, minerals, trace elements, amino acids, and so on, the pancreas (along with other parts of the body) suffers from this stress load, and malfunctions occur in the equipment. The names commonly used to refer to these malfunctions in the pancreas are hypoglycemia and diabetes. These two seemingly separate metabolic problems are basically only different stages of a more fundamental disease process, which will be discussed in greater detail in chapter 10.

There is evidence that all endocrine glands can be influenced by reactions to foods, chemicals, and/or inhalants.[58] These influences are usually in the nature of inhibition of function, as with the pancreas. Women in the involutional period characteristically lose their hot flashes, and libido improves in men and women, when there is proper avoidance and rotation of symptom-incriminated allergic substances. Low thyroid function characteristically returns to normal when avoiding and spacing of symptom-producing substances is practiced. In fact, the clinical impression is gained that primary endocrine disorders cannot be correctly assessed until after the removal of or nonsymptom-level spacing of all addictive substances.

For now, however, let us center our attention on the organ which encounters stress first and most drastically: the pancreas.

Reduced pancreatic function based on stress factors such as addictions, chemical toxins, and allergies, as well as established nutritional deficiencies, should be considered as the foundation on which many different degenerative diseases are built. A few consequences of the pancreatic deficiency process are:

1. a disordered acid base balance;
2. diminished pancreatic proteolytic enzyme levels in the blood;
3. digestive failure, resulting in a poor breakdown of proteins into amino acids;
4. the resulting circulation in the blood of nonusable proteins and peptides, which lodge in tissues and evoke kinin-inflammatory reactions; and
5. circulation in the blood of partially digested lipids.

Let us examine each of these consequences in more detail.

When too much stress causes the pancreas to function improperly, there is first a reduction in the proper levels of pancreatic bicarbonate. Bicarbonate is that pancreatic secretion that creates a necessary alkaline medium for the small intestine. In pancreatic deficiencies, acute metabolic acidosis usually occurs after the meal because the pancreatic bicarbonate now undersupplied has not neutralized the acid from the stomach as it empties into the duodenum. This reduction of proper bicarbonate levels results in a chain reaction whereby the pancreatic proteolytic enzymes, which need an alkaline medium in which to function best, are destroyed. Low production of pancreatic proteolytic enzymes, in turn, has the following consequences: amino-acid deficiency due to a lack of digestion of proteins to amino acids; poorly digested and undigested proteins being absorbed into the blood through the intestinal mucous membrane and evoking kinin-inflammatory reactions throughout the body; and a continual rise in kinin-inflammatory reactions in various tissue and organ targets. More specifically, a low level of the pancreatic enzymes chymotrypsin and carboxypeptidase in the blood allows the levels of the tissue hormone kinins to rise; this, in turn, evokes inflammatory reactions in different tissues and organs. Thus, once there is an inhibition of pancreatic function, and especially the pancreatic bicarbonate, there follows a chain reaction of inflammatory reactions throughout the body (including the brain) due to the fact that these all-important inflammation-controlling enzymes are in low supply. Undoubtedly, the majority of inflammatory reactions in mentally oriented degenerative diseases, especially schizophrenia, are kinin-evoked.

It is important to remember that when the pancreas is functioning poorly, in addition to a disordered acid-base balance and the resulting increase of nonusable and sometimes toxic protein particles (peptides) circulating in the blood, there is always an accompanying amino-acid deficiency. An amino-acid deficiency is a very serious problem because the central nervous system, as well as many other biochemical systems within the human body, malfunctions when there is a short supply of these necessary nutrients—the very building blocks of life.

A further problem related to pancreatic insufficiency is the lowered lipase activity it causes. Schizophrenics have been observed to have a characteristically higher than normal level of free fatty acids (lipids) in the blood. In a group of allergic, behaviorally disordered adolescents in whom about one-third had been psychotic, lipid metabolism was demonstrated to be abnormally high by studying phospholipid-cholesterol ratios. It is thought that this disordered phospholipid-cholesterol ratio reflects cell membrane instability, which may cause the cell to react more sensitively to allergic foods and chemicals. It has been postulated that there are two sources for this disordered lipid metabolism: reduced lipase enzyme production by the pancreas, lipase being the enzyme needed for proper lipid or fat metabolism; and a high-fat diet. It has been clinically observed that a low-fat diet, in place of the usual high-fat diet of our modern society, intervenes favorably in the degenerative disease process. Therefore, it appears logical that in cases in which lipase activity is low, one should reduce the fat intake in the diet as well as supplement it with not only pancreatic lipase enzymes but also a full spectrum of pancreatic proteolytic protein enzymes and bicarbonate.

In summary, the degenerative disease process develops in the following manner: chronic addictive reactions and their counterpart allergic reactions to foods, chemicals, and inhalants are the central stress factors, along with nutrient deficiencies in the diet that produce the pancreatic-deficiency disease process. Once the pancreas begins to function poorly, we encounter an acute metabolic acidosis occurring in the small intestine. This reduction of pancreatic bicarbonate destroys proteolytic enzymes; a lowered proteolytic enzyme level in the small intestine creates amino-acid deficiencies while the low proteolytic level in the blood allows a continual rise in kinin-inflammatory reactions to occur in various tissues and organs. Moreover, pancreatic insufficiency is responsible for a lowered lipase activity. A lower level of this enzyme appearing in the blood may cause metabolic activity at the cellular level to react in a more sensitive fashion to allergic foods and chemicals. The degenerative disease process now begins, and if it continues for any protracted period, these multiple deficiencies feed upon one another and add to the additional metabolic stress that finally breaks up the entire biochemical balance needed for health.

The far-reaching chain reaction of metabolic malfunctions set in motion by this disease process is staggering to contemplate. Kinin reactions in the brain alone have been clinically observed to fall into the classic psychiatric degenerative diagnostic categories of schizophrenia, manic depression, psychotic depression, hyperkinesis, autism, learning disabilities, hallucinations, delusions, and a host of others. The implications of these discoveries are numerous. Psychiatrists, neurologists, and physicians are now faced with the evidence that it is not just hallucinations, delusions, depressions, agitation, or other less severe reactions such as anxiety, headaches, and compulsions that they are dealing with, but a basic organic disease process with the consequences of numerous metabolic deficiencies, toxicities, addictions, and so forth, impinging on central-nervous-system function. To consider all these apparently different states in terms of a single disease process provides a valuable framework for treatment, whether the presenting symptomatology be mental or physical. Treating the basic underlying disease process rationally offers a much better prospect of achieving a final and lasting success than does the use of traditional methods. Of course, such treatment is possible only if psychiatrists and neurologists undertake a new approach to diagnosis, enlarging its scope to include a search for the evidence and causes of this disease process.

There is a great deal more to the degenerative disease process than I have been able to discuss here, but this brief summary emphasizes the fact that we need a new orientation, a new direction of research in which underlying metabolic degenerative disease processes are looked at in great detail and with continuing clinical interest.

I have concentrated on the pancreas, but it certainly is not the only endocrine gland significantly involved in the degenerative disease process. The adrenal gland, with its sixty or more corticosteroid hormones, is very important in handling stress; of course, each gland has its necessary function. There is evidence pointing to the clinical conclusion that the stress factors of maladaptive reactions to foods and chemicals produce a state that alters the normal processes of all the glands; this state is called a "panendocrine disorder." It can be related to either an over or underproduction of hormones. We have clinically recorded, for example, low adrenocortical hormones (adrenal gland), high progesterone production (ovaries), low thyroxine levels (thyroid gland), and low estrogen production (ovaries) in response to maladaptive allergic reactions. The causes of these disorders, along with all the other interactions between them, need to be studied further.

It is time for medicine to recognize that more research needs to be directed at the nutritional orthomolecular-ecologic problems which develop at the cellular level. No longer can we be content merely to treat symptoms. We must direct our attention toward the prevention and treatment of degenerative disease by studying and using those substances that normally occur in the human body. Then and only then will we be able to understand the total disease process.

Maladaptive allergic and addictive food and chemical reactions in most cases bear a direct relationship to a nutritionally deficient state. More specifically, because the frequent use of only a few foods uses up specific enzymes needed for metabolism, and also fails to provide the necessary broad spectrum of nutrients demanded by proper metabolism, such a diet may help to create a nutritionally deficient state within certain cells, tissues, and organs of the body. The chronic use of substances making unusual demands on body chemistry (e.g., tea, coffee, alcohol, tobacco), or chronic contact with pollutants such as gas fumes, insecticide residues, industrial wastes, lead, mercury, or the like, or the continual intake of food colorings and additives all drain the body of nutrients necessary to cellular metabolism. The specific tissues in which a nutritional deficiency is occurring often can give us a clue as to the specific nutrient in low supply. For example, inadequate amounts of vitamins A and D produce unhealthy and therefore overreactive mucous membranes. Deficiencies of the B-complex, and especially B_6, and of vitamin C produce unhealthy brain function and predispose patients to maladaptive reactions of the central nervous system. The same is true for minerals; magnesium, for instance, is one of the most important elements for healthy brain function, and its presence at less than optimal levels can have serious consequences.

What specific effect, then, do these states of nutritional deficiency have on the proper functioning of our body's metabolism? The answer to this question is important, for it will give us deeper insights into the relationships existing between these deficiency states and the disease process previously discussed.

It has been clinically observed that maladaptive reactions to foods, chemicals, and inhalants most often produce localized inflammatory edema and toxicity in specific target tissues and/or organs of the body. This reaction compromises the healthy functioning of the local tissues in several ways. First, associated with kinin-mediated, inflammatory, allergic edema is an often severely lowered oxygen level in the specific reacting tissue. This results in cellular injury, which makes further demands for specific nutrients already in short supply. Such a vicious cycle of nutritional deficiencies, allergic response, localized edema, cellular injury associated with lower levels of oxygen supply, and consequently even greater nutritional deficiencies encourages locally present and usually dormant opportunist, infectious microorganisms to become active. To put it another way, each time there exists an acute allergic reaction resulting from a nutritional deficiency, no matter what the specific reaction is, there simultaneously exists an inflammatory edema causing a local reduction in oxygen supply to tissues involved in the reaction. Once this has occurred, a favorable biological state exists for a flare-up of infection. Infectious microorganisms quickly multiply at staggering rates and become toxin-producing. This infectious toxicity causes the biochemical system to become even more nutritionally deficient, and the end result is a low level of immunological defense, which invites even more infectious invasion, since proper levels of antibodies used in the fight against infections cannot be attained unless optimum nutrition is available; a more severe allergic sensitivity also results.

We can see, therefore, that the disease process is a chain reaction, with each state bringing about the next. This biochemical chain reaction is so tightly interrelated that one cannot speak of one link in the chain without considering its place in the whole chain. The disease process must be thought of as a dynamic process involving many different yet interdependent and interacting aspects. It is thus not advisable to center one's attention on symptomatic treatment and relief of one part of the disease process. All the dynamics involved must be taken into consideration and acted upon accordingly.

Infections are one of the very important links in our biochemical disease-process chain; let us examine for a moment some interesting discoveries concerning them. Schizophrenics, like other organically ill patients, harbor multiple infectious agents that can become active at any time in their lives. Clinical experience has demonstrated cultures of ten to fifteen different types of infections from schizophrenics; in one specific case, twenty-nine infections including bacteria and fungi were discovered. It is important not only that these infections do indeed exist, but also that mental symptoms can at times be produced by reexposure to these infectious agents. One twenty-four-year-old schizophrenic, for example, developed acute catatonia on a single exposure to *Candida albicans.* But what is even more interesting is that she had a history of episodic *Candida albicans* vaginal infections. Another example is that of an eighteen-year-old paranoid schizophrenic who had nasal staphylococcus infections many times in his life. He became paranoid and developed a stuffy nose when sublingually tested with staphylococcus vaccine.

Based on clinical evidence, we can now say that many different infectious microorganisms can be demonstrated to be as powerful toxic agents in producing specific maladaptive reactions as specific foods, chemicals, and inhalants. Therefore, the infections the patient is harboring should always be a part of the differential diagnosis that points to the various causes of symptoms. Also, it is probably true that there are no tissues or organs in the human body free from an assortment of varying types of latent opportunist microorganisms. In fact, we must consider it probable that one of the final deteriorating processes in organic disease is that of microbial invasion, with the resultant tissue damage and toxins interfering with the patient's nutritional, hormonal, and enzymatic systems. Every attempt should be made to eliminate the environment by which these microorganisms can become active and multiply.

One aspect of treatment which centers on infectious microorganisms is reinforcement of the immunological defenses. The three key words for this approach are *vaccination, nutrition,* and *avoidance.*

The first step is the use of autogenous vaccines composed of bodies of the microorganisms and/or their toxins, isolated from the blood or urine. Such vaccines can also be made from cultures from infections sited in the skin, ear, nose, throat, mouth, and armpits. It does not matter from which source the vaccine is made, but only that it is made from the patient's own microorganism population, hence the term *autogenous* ("self-born"). In spite of all the many infections cultured from schizophrenics, there is only one organism that has been observed to be characteristically present in all cases. That organism is *Progenitor cryptocides.* Two stock vaccines (i.e., vaccines that are not made from the patient's own body fluids) important in this case are BCG and Maruyama. The former is derived from *Mycobacterium tuberculosis,* the latter from *Mycobacterium leprae.* Both these vaccines have a cross-antigenicity with *Progenitor cryptocides,* as they all belong to the order *Actinomycetales.* Other stock vaccines that have varying degrees of usefulness in stimulating immunologic defenses are sheep cell, flu vaccine, poison ivy-oak-sumac, and stock respiratory bacterial vaccines.

Second, there needs to be optimum nutrition. This means an optimum supply of amino acids and specific minerals as well as all the vitamins, especially vitamins C, B_6, and pantothenic acid, which are needed to support adrenocortical function during the stress of vaccination as well as optimum white-blood-cell proliferation. Antibodies cannot be formed unless there is an optimum supply of these three nutrients, as well as an adequate supportive base of all the other necessary nutrients.

Minerals are far more important in this respect than once thought. Hair biopsy (analysis) sometimes reveals either specific mineral deficiencies, which can be easily corrected with appropriate supplements, or occasional evidence of toxic levels of lead, mercury, cadmium, nickel, tin, or aluminum. These mineral toxicities not only interfere with proper central-nervous-system function, but can also deplete the system of other nutritional factors, establishing a fertile environment in which infectious microorganisms can flourish. Mineral toxicity usually is related to individual habits, which must be explored and, if necessary, corrected. For example, eating large quantities of tuna often provides an excess of cadmium; cooking with aluminum utensils can cause toxic levels of that metal to appear in the body; some hair dyes contain very large amounts of lead, which can be absorbed through the scalp; and drinking water may contain one or more toxic metals. Therefore, any orthomolecular-ecologic profile study of immunological defenses must include consideration of the presence and sources of toxic metals.

Third, we must establish an optimum local and systemic cellular function by avoidance, spacing of contact, and rotation of allergy-incriminating foods, chemicals, and inhalants. These three principles must be honored or allergic reactions will begin to appear. Once this happens, you have kinin-mediated inflammation in specific target tissues and the resultant reduction of oxygen levels. When there are low oxygen levels, there are much greater chances of a flare-up of infectious microorganisms.

This three-part approach to dealing with infection is obviously more complicated and time-consuming than the familiar practice of administering antibiotics. However, while antibiotics may temporarily stop the spread of infectious microorganisms, their use does not improve the nutritionally weak biochemical situation, ameliorate the addictive food reactions associated with nutritional deficiencies, or bolster the failing immunological defense system, which allowed the infection to occur in the first place. As a result, the likelihood that infections will continue to poison the system is very great. To be sure, symptomatic treatment may stop one or more infectious flare-ups, but the degenerative disease process continues uninterrupted.

The same is true for symptomatic therapy of allergically mediated kinin-inflammatory reactions. A specific phenothiazine may reduce an allergic reaction and thus temporarily stop a particular undesirable symptom; but again, the underlying disease process continues. This may result later in more severe nutritional deficiencies, greater susceptibility to infectious invasion, more cerebral allergies, and a four-to-five times greater chance of becoming diabetic or developing permanent Parkinson's disease or tardive dyskinesia. I want to emphasize that unless the etiology—the root cause—of the entire disease process is first clinically discovered and then treated via orthomolecular-ecologic methods, dire results will almost certainly be produced by symptomatic treatment methods.

In spite of numerous observations over the years of mental and physical reactions to foods, chemicals, inhalants, microorganisms, and the symptom consequences of nutritional deficiencies and infections, heavy metal toxicity, and the biological consequences of allergy and addiction, it is not popular to seriously consider these factors in the differential diagnosis of mental and emotional illness; they are usually only slightly considered in chronic physical degenerative diseases. There are indications that the widespread determination to ignore the evidence supporting the concepts of orthomolecular-ecologic diagnosis and treatment of mental illness is weakening. Many physicians and patients experienced in current traditional psychiatric diagnosis and treatment are gratified by the results obtained by this approach to diagnosis and treatment. What I have been discussing is not a miracle cure, but rather an abundantly healthy lifestyle that must be unqualifiedly adopted if the person is to be symptom-free or relatively so. This altered way of life offers the prospect of stopping, and to some degree even reversing, the progress of chronic physical and mental degenerative diseases. The present evidence clearly shows the need for long-term, intense—and necessarily expensive—scientific evaluations of clinical orthomolecular-ecologic medicine as applied to chronic degenerative diseases in general and psychosis in particular.

The most profitable approach to discovering the sources of acute and chronic degenerative disease, whether physical or mental, is to examine broadly the body chemistry and function during a symptom-reduced or symptom-free state occurring after a four-to-six-day period of avoidance of symptom-incriminated substances; this then should be compared with the abnormal chemical shifts and disordered functions appearing in the symptom-evoked state occurring during allergy testing of single substance exposures. Such a method does not violate Roger J. Williams's principle of "biochemical individuality," since each patient is tested on an individual basis. The patient's unique biochemical pattern is analyzed and compared before and after allergy-testing procedures. That is, the patient's condition is not compared to someone else's disordered biochemistry; she is studied as a functioning individual with specific needs, deficiencies, and unique biochemical problems. The patient serves as her own control. Thus, without double-blind studies on hundreds of cases, we have believable evidence of a cause-and-effect relationship existing between stimulus and response before and after testing. This basic method has been recommended and profitably applied by many physicians.

In this and previous chapters, we have discussed at length the purely physical components of what traditional medical doctrine regards as mental and emotional conditions. We hope and believe that we have presented sufficient evidence to convince the lay or professional reader that nutritional deficiencies, allergic-addictive reactions, and their effects on the system are strongly implicated in degenerative conditions, whether of the mind or the body. We do not, however, wish to give the impression that conventional psychiatric techniques and methods are irrelevant or unimportant. Even if the physical aspect of the degenerative process is effectively dealt with, there remains a residuum of maladaptive learned responses, lack of maturity, and deficiency in social responses produced by illness; this requires treatment in terms of psychology rather than physiology.

Therefore, there are three elements to be considered in differential diagnosis:

1. symptoms as an expression of nutritional deficiencies or excesses, or heavy metal toxicity
2. symptoms as an expression of a reaction to environmental substances such as foods, chemicals, inhalants, and microorganisms and their toxins
3. symptoms as learned responses to life experiences

The most satisfactory treatment format is that which takes into account all these factors. Orthomolecular medicine was established to diagnose and treat symptoms in terms of deficiency and toxicity. Ecologic medicine examines and deals with symptoms as reactions to substances. Avoidance of symptom-incriminated substances has more immediate clinical value than giving a nutrient or removing a toxic heavy metal; the detection and treatment of both ecologic and metabolic factors gives increased values beyond either approach alone. In fact, satisfactory clinical results frequently cannot be achieved unless these two systems are combined. Therefore, orthomolecular-ecologic medicine is not rapidly developing in the direction of further study of how nutritional factors and ecologic controls affect each other. Physicians who combine orthomolecular medicine with human ecology are discovering that optimum successful treatment involves a simultaneous combination of:

1. an initial three-month avoidance of allergy-producing, incriminated substances;
2. a four-day rotation of foods with the reinstatement of incriminated foods in three months if they are still not symptom-producing;
3. specific appropriate treatment for laboratory-demonstrated deficiencies: vitamins C, B_1, B_3, B_6, B_{12}, folic acid, amino acids, minerals, lead, mercury, cadmium, nickel, and so on;
4. general supportive nutrition, including diet and nutrient supplements to meet all individually determined cellular needs;
5. supporting pancreatic function with enzymes and amino acids in those patients who do not completely reinstate its function after a period of time;
6. vigorous exercise; and
7. psychological treatment such as training down phobias and obsessions and compulsions, problem solving and teaching of social skills and personality maturity.

This orthomolecular-ecologic metabolic profile applies equally to chronic physical and chronic mental illnesses.

It has been traditional, and in many respects useful, for medical science to define sharply the differences in diseases. However, it should now be clear that it is also important and profitable to diagnose and treat the chronic degenerative disease process, which is a common factor in both physical and mental diseases. This approach provides the measures by which a physician can take steps to halt and, to some degree, reverse the degenerative disease process.

Chapter 9

Preventive Self-Help

We stated earlier that nutritional treatment of the conditions discussed in this book is a matter for professionals, and the research and case histories presented as evidence for the conclusions drawn have all been taken from professional sources. Yet a book such as this, intended to acquaint the lay public as well as the concerned physician with the concepts of orthomolecular medicine and human ecology, should present some information that the individual reader can use to advantage; there are certain measures such a reader may take that can promote better health or enhance his understanding of his basic mental and physical condition, especially with regard as to what type of professional assistance might be sought.

No two people have exactly the same inherited characteristics carried in his or her body's estimated 100,000 genes. Therefore, no two people have the same nutrient needs. Some may need meganutrient doses, while others may need only micronutrient doses. In other words, the dosage of a specific nutrient or group of nutrients that will help with one individual may be too low or too high for another individual. Keeping this thought in mind, and also the fact that all nutrients work together as a team, Roger J. Williams, Ph.D., has formulated a basic "health insurance" program that most people can adopt as a preventive measure. This formula, coupled with the rotation diet, will supply for everyone a degree of protection against developing allergic or addictive responses to foods and chemicals. He suggests the following daily dosages:

Vitamin A	7,500 IU
Vitamin D	400 IU
Vitamin E	40 IU
Vitamin K	2 mg
Vitamin C	250 mg
Vitamin B_1	2 mg
Vitamin B_2	2 mg
Vitamin B_6	3 mg
Vitamin B_{12}	9 mg
Niacinamide	20 mg
Pantothenic acid	15 mg
Biotin	0.3 mg
Folic acid	0.4 mg
Choline	250 mg
Inositol	250 mg
Para-aminobenzoic acid (PABA)	30 mg
Rutin	200 mg
Calcium	750 mg
Phosphate	750 mg
Magnesium	200 mg
Iron	15 mg
Zinc	15 mg
Copper	2 mg
Iodine	0.15 mg
Manganese	5 mg
Molybdenum	0.1 mg
Chromium	1.0 mg
Selenium	0.02 mg
Cobalt	0.1 mg

However, if chronic physical or mental problems do continue, it might be advisable to consult an orthomolecular-ecologic physician who is trained to administer megaformulations of nutrients and will probably use some or all of the following nutrients in varying dosages. Of course, different physicians throughout the country may want to raise or lower the following megadoses depending upon the patient and the specific problem being treated.

Variations of Meganutrient Formulations Per Day

Vitamin A	10,000	to	50,000 IU
Vitamin B_1	50	to	1,500 mg
Vitamin B_2	50	to	1,500 mg
Vitamin B_6	50	to	1,500 mg
Vitamin B_{12}	500	to	3,000 mcg
Niacin	100	to	1,500 mg
Biotin	0.3	to	0.6 mg
Choline	250	to	1,000 mg
Folic acid	1	to	5 mg
Inositol	500	to	1,000 mg
Para-aminobenzoic acid (PABA)	300	to	1,500 mg
Pantothenic acid	100	to	1,500 mg
Vitamin C	1,000	to	10,000 mg or higher
Vitamin D	400	to	1,200 IU
Vitamin E	400	to	2,400 IU
Calcium	500	to	1,000 mg
Magnesium	100	to	300 mg
Iron	20	to	60 mg
Iodine	150	to	300 mcg
Copper	5	to	15 mg
Zinc	15	to	30 mg
Chromium	1	to	3 mg
Manganese	5	to	15 mg
Selenium	200 mcg		

These lists of nutrients do not mention any specific amino acids, enzymes, or hormones that might also be used by a physician treating particular medical problems. However, since it has been reported that chronic degenerative diseases, whether physical or mental, to a large degree relate to the chronic stress of addiction and similar reactive states, it is preferable that a physician be the one to sort out the reactions to foods and chemicals, test for infections and other specific nutritionally related deficiencies, and treat the patient accordingly.

Unfortunately, many people who are really quite ill, especially emotionally ill, have a misconception that they can do all this on their own. In trying to have people help themselves when they have insisted on doing it themselves, I have run into the unhappy situation of patients claiming that the system did not work, when in reality they had never followed it closely enough to give it a chance. I have thus become disillusioned about emotionally and mentally ill patients helping themselves. I feel that they really should have professional help. It is possible that they may react to a food and have such serious symptoms as to require immediate professional help. In short, there are many people who should not attempt self-help, and there is no way for a doctor to know who these people are unless he examines them. Therefore, anyone engaging in self-help must do so without considering it as a prescription from a doctor. It is equally important that this book not be misconstrued as a prescription for self-help. Some people can fast for a period of four to five days without any problems. Others will have very serious complications. Some might experience such severe depression that they wish to die. Others might have seizures or asthmatic attacks. Still others will crash directly into a full-blown psychosis. It should be pointed out that it is not absolutely necessary to fast. Foods that are seldom used can be taken instead. These should be foods that do not relate even family-wise to the foods that that person commonly uses. However, this does not assure the patient that he will not have adverse reactions to the foods to which he is addicted and which he is now withdrawing from his diet. Again, caution is the important word in dealing with any of these matters.

Obviously, there are still large numbers of people who are capable of self-assessment without either physical or emotional danger. These people can receive considerable benefits just by being oriented to the material in this book.

The pulse test is one possible instrument for self-help and recognition of allergies. If the pulse is within the normal range before the suspected food is eaten, it should be taken every fifteen to thirty minutes for about one and a half hours after the food is eaten. A pulse rate above 84 (in the high 80s or 90s or beyond) at this point is usually indicative of allergic reactions. Occasionally the opposite is true, with the pulse markedly decreasing, giving a brachycardia (slow heart action) instead of a tachycardia (rapid heart action). This is also indicative of possible allergic reactions.

The pulse test picks up only a few of the maladaptive reactions. However, there is another technique for self-detection of allergic reactions. This method involves using a long-wave ultraviolet light shone on a test tube of urine. To do this, fill the test tube three-quarters full and shine the light downward at a 45 degree angle, making sure the test tube has no gummed stickers on it as they will cause an abnormal shine. The normal color for urine is a straw or clear color. Often the urine will turn blue (any shade from light to dark) after an allergic reaction. Occasionally the urine will turn pink or even deep red. These pink-red colors indicate porphyria, which seldom occurs, but it is also connected with allergic reactions. Test the urine before the food is eaten; if it is normal, then proceed with the food; three hours later test the urine again. If there are any samples that of necessity are urinated before that time, test these also. However, the three-hour level is when reactions are most likely to show up. These long-wave ultraviolet lights (commonly called black lights) are inexpensive and can be purchased from any medical supply house. Doctors often use them to look at fungus infections.

A technique of monitoring for allergic reactions that we use constantly in the office is to examine the blood sugar one hour after each test meal. If the person is diabetic, it should be tested before and one hour after the test meal. However, if it is beyond 160 milligrams percent with a test meal, it is always tested again before the next meal to make sure that it has normalized down to 115 milligrams percent or less. This requires more skill since pricking the finger with a small lance is necessary. The instrument used is an Eyetone machine with a Dextrostix. Several drops of blood are placed on a Dextrostix and allowed to set for one minute, then washed off. This, in turn, is placed in the meter and read. The Eyetone instrument is made by the Miles Laboratory Company and can be purchased from medical supply companies. They will also instruct the person in its use and in the fingerpricking technique. Blood sugars that are 160 milligrams percent and beyond are significant and represent an allergic, diabetic-related reaction.

Chapter 10

Diabetes and Hypoglycemia: *A New Look at an Old Problem*

Diabetes and hypoglycemia are usually thought of as distinct disease entities calling for specific treatment. The purpose of this chapter is to show that, on the contrary, these conditions are aspects of the degenerative disease process discussed in the preceding chapter, and to demonstrate approaches to diagnosis and treatment based on this concept.

The proper maintenance of constant and adequate glucose (blood sugar) levels in the body is one of the most important functions of our biochemical being. Our brain needs glucose in order to think clearly; our muscles need glucose for strength and action; our entire bodies need glucose to maintain life. A delicately regulated process of the body ensures that we have proper levels of glucose in our blood. The anterior pituitary gland, which produces hormones that elevate blood sugar; the adrenal medulla, which produces epinephrine (adrenalin) that stimulates the breakdown of stored glycogen (carbohydrate stored in the liver); and the adrenal cortex, which produces a number of hormones called glucosteroids that are necessary for the metabolism of all carbohydrates simultaneously act like instruments in a harmonious and complex symphony of metabolism so that an adequate level of glucose can be supplied to the body. The pancreas, in turn, produces insulin, which regulates the level of blood sugar and thus helps to control any diabetic symptoms.

Figure 10.1 illustrates varying degrees of abnormal blood-sugar levels. For example, line A is diabetes, in which there is an insufficient amount of insulin in the blood, and the blood sugar level is obviously too high. Line B shows a very sudden drop in proper sugar levels (i.e., hypoglycemia) from 220 to 80 after the first half hour. In testing for hypoglycemia, the speed of the drop is an important diagnostic tool. This is what Alan Nittler, M.D., had in mind

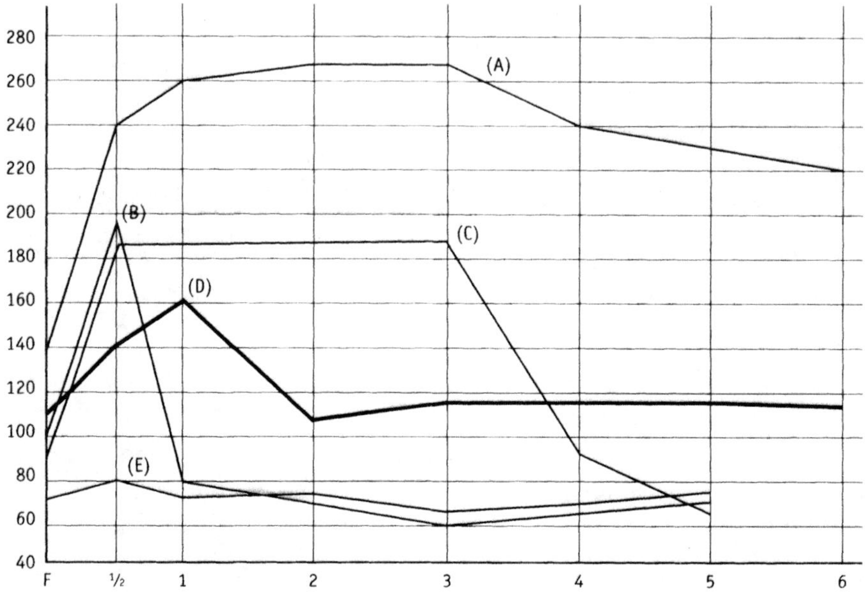

FIGURE 10.1. *Abnormal Glucose Tolerance Tests*

Line A: Diabetes (high blood sugar)

Line B: Early Hypoglycemia (low blood sugar). A very sudden and precipitous drop coming after only one-half hour of testing.

Line C: Late Hypoglycemia coming in the third or fourth hour.

Line D: Functional Hypoglycemia. A drop in the 40 to 50 range like this can cause convulsions.

Line E: Flat Curve Hypoglycemia, usually accompanied by a flat emotional response and a tired feeling all the time.

when he listed his five criteria for the interpretation of the five-hour, seven-specimen test. They are:

1. The blood-glucose level must rise to the half-hour and on up to the one-hour level (solid black line in Figure 10.1). In other words, there must be at least one hour of increased energy because of the glucose intake.
2. The percentage differential between the fasting and the lowest sugar levels must not exceed 20 percent. There must be low-level stability in order to prevent the low symptomatic points.
3. There must be no levels lower than the normal low level established for the test used. If the test used states 70 to 110 as the normal range, then there should be no levels below 70 milligrams percent.
4. The drop from the high point to the low should be about 50 milligrams percent. A steep and precipitous drop adds to the stress of life.
5. The one-hour level must be at least 50 percent greater than the fasting level.

A positive diagnosis of hypoglycemia can be made if any one of these criteria is positive. This must be qualified since a diabetic curve can be positive in the third criterion and not be hypoglycemia. However, there are many cases that are diabetic in the first hours only to become hypoglycemic in the later hours. The significant fact is that, for our purposes, any variation from the solid "normal line pattern" in Figure 10.1 should be considered as a sign of either hypoglycemia (low blood sugar) or hyperglycemia (high blood sugar).[59]

There are various symptoms that may or may not occur when there is a rapid rise or fall in the blood sugar:

MENTAL SYMPTOMS
confusion, forgetfulness, difficulty concentrating, mind goes blank

EMOTIONAL SYMPTOMS
emotional instability, strong temper, impatience and irritability, depression, uncontrollable crying spells

PHYSICAL SYMPTOMS
Vision: blurred, double vision, sensitivity to light

Pains: headaches, aching joints and twitching muscles, weakness, mental confusion after physical or emotional stress

Related illness: allergies or asthma, alcoholism, susceptibility to infectious diseases, emotional instability

Time of symptoms: feelings of weakness and irritability in the morning before breakfast; other symptoms can occur generally two or more hours after eating or after exhausting physical or emotional stress.[60]

For many years, there has existed in medicine a generalization relating to carbohydrate intolerance. The diabetic and hypoglycemic are said to have carbohydrate intolerance because of the fact that a single carbohydrate (corn sugar) food test with blood-sugar levels monitored before and after the test meal (as in Figure 10.1) offers evidence that a patient cannot properly handle sugar. Having accepted this idea, one may conclude that the blood sugar is either too high or too low because of carbohydrate intolerance. From this evidence it is also assumed that all other carbohydrates will not be tolerated. Treatment of these carbohydrate-intolerance conditions logically involves reducing carbohydrate intake.

However, there are physicians who have discovered that hypoglycemia and hyperglycemia can be evoked in a person who has ingested any food or come in contact with any chemical to which she is allergic. Broad-spectrum food and chemical symptom-induction testing, with blood sugar and pH monitored before and after the test, reveal the surprising fact that low and high blood sugar can be evoked by foods of *all* types, whether fats, carbohydrates, or proteins, and that chemicals such as petrochemical hydrocarbons and even tobacco equally evoke abnormal sugar level curves in susceptible persons. The foods causing these reactions are specific for each person. Carbohydrates predominate as symptom-precipitating substances, but the reactions are not limited to carbohydrates and can be caused by any substance to which the person reacts maladaptively. The simple fact of the matter is that abnormal sugar levels in the body are caused by allergic-like reactions to specific substances. The central problem in hypoglycemia and diabetes is not that of a general type of food (i.e., carbohydrates) but that of an individual maladaptive allergic reaction, which in turn interferes with proper blood sugar levels. These maladaptive reactions must always be individually diagnosed by provocative food testing.

In short, hypoglycemia and hyperglycemia should not be considered strictly in terms of carbohydrate metabolism dysfunction. Rather, clinically suspected, incriminating substances of all kinds must be examined in light of allergic biochemical individuality and treatment administered accordingly.

Case histories

A thirty-year-old man appeared as a manic-depressive reaction, depressive type, with episodic psychotic degrees of depression including a suicide attempt and dissociated episodes during which time he went places and did things of which he had no memory. As an infant, he was diagnosed as having a milk allergy and of necessity used soy milk instead of cow's milk. As an adult, he assumed he had outgrown his milk allergy and daily used dairy products in large quantities.

He was symptom-free by the fourth day of the fast, using non-chemically treated water only. A test meal of pasteurized milk plunged him into the depths of depression. Blood-sugar level was normal before and after the test. His symptoms were relieved by the following intravenous nutrients: 12.5 grams of vitamin C and 20 cc of adrenocortical extract (double strength). Powdered skim milk, cheddar cheese, and American cheese gave no symptoms. With Swiss cheese, he was cold and sweaty. Butter evoked a severe depression. Cream cheese was a favorite food, which he frequently used. He also loved and frequently used a blue-cheese dressing containing cream cheese. Before the test for cream cheese began, he was symptom-free, but within fifteen minutes of the test meal, symptoms began to develop. At first he felt like withdrawing from other people due to a contemplative and depressive feeling. Within another fifteen minutes, he was severely depressed and withdrew from the hospital parlor to the seclusion of his room. He was over-reacting to sounds and sights and would cringe as if afraid of being attacked. At this point, half an hour after the test meal, he was dissociated and later had no memory of what happened around him. Two hours after the test meal, he was alternately experiencing extreme fright at environmental stimuli, with no verbal communication, and a comatose state of no response to sight and sound stimuli. He was fluctuating between a pulse rate of 123 and blood pressure of 170/110 and a pulse of 50 and blood pressure of 114/50. At this point his blood sugar was 20 milligrams percent. It was difficult to believe, so the test was run four times with the same result. He was given 12.5 grams of vitamin C, 1,000 milligrams of B_6, 10 cc of calcium gluconate, 2 grams of magnesium sulfate, and 20 cc of adrenocortical extract (double strength). With this he awakened, was communicative, understood, and was not frightened by environmental stimuli. He was too weak to stand and had a pounding headache. His pulse was 80 and blood pressure 130/84. He was given 50 mE1 of sodium bicarbonate intravenously and his headache left. He was still too weak to stand, and he complained of spots and indistinct vision. His blood sugar was again taken and found to be 30 milligrams percent. He was given 6 teaspoons of beet sugar, a glass of pineapple juice, and several bites of chocolate cake. Prior testing had demonstrated him not to be symptom-reactive to cereal grains, beet, or pineapple. Within thirty minutes, his blood sugar was 160 milligrams percent and he was symptom-free aside from an apprehension for several hours that the symptom state could suddenly return.

The above described hypoglycemia occurring in response to a food test is the most severe and most prolonged ever observed in our clinic. The assumption that these disordered reactions will be in response to carbohydrate only is not valid. Testing reveals that they occur with any type of food, and that the central cause is the state of being allergic to or allergic in a specific way to a specific food (fat, protein, or carbohydrate) or chemical. In the previously mentioned case history, the hypoglycemic response was to cream cheese, which is largely a protein and fat food.

A forty-five-year-old man had a morning fasting blood sugar of 250 milligrams percent. He had already been studied by an allergist, and his food and chemical allergies were known. His potential to develop diabetes mellitus (hyperglycemia) had not been assessed since this is not a routine in allergy assessments. The goal was to discover a way to increase his ability to rotate a reasonable number of foods into his four-day, food-rotation program. Foods were chosen for testing that he had not eaten for several days. All foods were withheld until his blood sugar was normal. This required sixteen hours' fasting.

He was symptom-free before the test meal of Irish potatoes, with blood sugar at 80 milligrams percent. Forty-five minutes after the test meal, his blood sugar was 280 milligrams percent; his symptoms were described as a spaced-out feeling and a sense of loss of balance, particularly when he walked.

An hour and a half before a second test meal, the following nutrients were given orally: 4 grams of vitamin C, 1,000 milligrams of B_6, 100 milligrams of B_1, 500 milligrams of niacinamide, 100 milligrams of B_2, 100 milligrams of pantothenic acid, 10,000 units of vitamin A, 800 units of vitamin E, 1 milligram of folic acid, 2.8 milligrams of manganese, 5 milligrams of zinc, 45 milligrams of magnesium, and 50 micrograms of chromium. He was symptom-free before the test meal, and his blood sugar was 60 milligrams percent. Before eating the potato he drank one tablespoon of safflower oil to reduce the absorption rate and thus reduce the allergic trigger mechanism. Forty-five minutes after the test meal, his blood sugar was 120 milligrams percent. No symptoms developed during the test!

This case illustrates the value of nutrients and oil before test meals. Selective trials with varying amounts of nutrients and oil led to the following conclusions:

1. The most important nutrient in relieving food-allergic symptoms is B_6, with vitamin C a good second, with the other nutrients subserving these two.
2. In a majority of reactions, the use of nutrients without the oil is successful.
3. Oil with or without nutrients is sometimes useful in reducing allergic reactions, probably due to its slowing of the absorption of foods, but it is not routinely used to reduce allergic reactions.

A twenty-five-year-old schizophrenic man was observed to be delusional and compulsively verbalizing his delusions after smoking a cigarette. He was also excessively hungry and thirsty. His morning fasting blood sugars were erratic, usually being about 100 milligrams percent, but on several occasions ranged between 200 to 300 milligrams percent. It was discovered that, when his fasting blood sugar was abnormally high, he was sneaking a cigarette before the test.

His fasting sugar was 75 milligrams percent, and he was symptom-free before the test. He smoked eight cigarettes in thirty minutes. During the test, he became delusional and compulsively verbalized his delusions, starting with the second cigarette. Thirty minutes after starting the smoking test, his blood sugar was 200 milligrams percent (hyperglycemia).

A twenty-four-year-old man was a three-pack-a-day cigarette smoker. He went twenty-four hours without smoking before a cigarette smoking test. His blood sugar was 80 milligrams percent before the test. With the first cigarette, he was sweating and was too weak to stand. Thirty minutes after the test began, his blood sugar was 30 milligrams percent (severe hypoglycemia).

It is obvious that these cases give convincing evidence that both hypoglycemia and hyperglycemia can be evoked by maladaptive reactions to tobacco even without the introduction of any foods. It has been observed clinically that petrochemical hydrocarbons such as exhaust fumes, perfumes, and gas stoves or heating units are equally potent sources in producing a disordered carbohydrate metabolism. Based on this evidence of allergy-evoked, carbohydrate-metabolism interference as the most frequent cause of hypoglycemia and hyperglycemia, it has been clinically demonstrated that the most effective treatment for this kind of disorder is avoidance of the incriminated foods and chemicals. In fact, some patients have been adequately managed by diet alone, including some who required insulin before allergy treatment.

It should now be clear that diabetes and hypoglycemia should be viewed as manifestations of the degenerative process explored in the preceding chapter, and that the chain reaction of maladaptive reaction, addiction, nutritional deficiency, weakened resistance to infection, and stress-related[61] breakdown of specific tissues and organs applies to these conditions just as much as to those previously described. The hyperglycemia (elevated blood sugar), which characterizes diabetes, can be considered as the exhaustion stage of the stress reaction, and hypoglycemia as the adaptation stage. Initial treatment for each condition should include identification of allergy-producing foods or substances, then avoidance and spacing. As with other degenerative disease manifestations, orthomolecular treatment will probably be required: vitamin and mineral supplementation, hormonal adjustment, and proteolytic-enzyme and amino-acid therapy. The general principles of this approach have been discussed in this chapter; a more detailed exposition of treatment and examination methods, of interest chiefly to physicians, is given in the appendix.

What should be emphasized here is that the orthomolecular-ecologic treatment of these complex and often painful conditions has been shown to be dramatically effective. One striking illustration of this is that, when this treatment method is followed, it has been our experience that the traditional insulin supplementation will be necessary in only the severest cases of maturity-onset diabetes mellitus instead of the majority. Treating rationally the basic underlying disease process with orthomolecular-ecologic techniques thus appears to present a much greater chance of success than other methods.

Success in the treatment of disease of all kinds is what every physician seeks in his practice. R. Glen Green, M.D., is a good example of a physician who learned how difficult it sometimes is to achieve this clinical goal, especially when the subject matter is hypo/hyperglycemia. The following account depicts Green's struggle in discovering a successful treatment modality for hypo/hyperglycemia. His search for clinical success was not an easy one, but his final realization of truth was well worth the struggle for himself as well as all his patients.

> By 1968, I was fed up with the way I was practicing medicine. I would go to the penitentiary nearly every morning, then to the hospitals for rounds and to do anesthesia or surgery. The afternoons were filled with patients whose complaints varied from day to day, from week to week. Neurotics seemed to be my lot. Just as I relieved a set of symptoms, another set popped up. Medicine was like a rotating squirrel's cage, and I was the squirrel. The harder I worked the more there was to do, all to little avail. The same patients kept returning endlessly, searching for answers, and I gave them more of the same medicine. . . .
>
> About this time, Dr. Hoffer's work was written up in *Maclean's,* a national magazine. His brand of psychiatry appealed to me. I arranged an apprenticeship with him in October of 1968. This was

the turning point for me in medicine and in my life. . . . It was about this time that my own allergy tolerance was exhausted. I began to suffer increasing fatigue and irritability. Instead of playing eighteen holes of golf I had to quit after eleven because I just couldn't swing the club. I needed more and more sleep, yet I was still tired. Eventually a glucose tolerance test (with corn sugar) was done. To my amazement, my curve went from 100 up to 212 in thirty minutes, then dropped rapidly to 80, then returned to the fasting level. Naturally, I read everything available on the subject. Traditional medical books and journals dismissed the subject of low blood sugar out of hand. If the sugar level was more than 50, there was no hypoglycemia. This led me to John Tintera's writings[62] and to medical meetings where doctors, who thought differently, would congregate. I started on the low-blood-sugar diet, then began to look for and find my symptoms in my patients. They, too, were sensitive to refined carbohydrates and had hypoglycemia. Throughout Tintera's writings, he frequently referred to allergy. I didn't twig to the importance of this until much later. I began to do five-hour sugar-tolerance curves on many of my patients. I used the hypoglycemic diet (i.e., high protein, moderate fat, and low carbohydrate) plus megadoses of vitamins C and B_3 to clear symptoms. Many patients, myself included, did well for a time.

In 1973, I attended a meeting in San Francisco at which Dr. Theron G. Randolph spoke about food allergy. I asked about hypoglycemia. He denied its existence. He claimed that hypoglycemia was merely an expression of food allergy, and the symptoms could be brought on by foods other than refined carbohydrates. By now I was getting up at night to eat peanuts and cheese or drink milk. Randolph laughed and said, "Exactly and what do you think that is—food allergy." I had to listen because my symptoms were coming back with a vengeance in spite of the low-blood-sugar diet. Now the jigsaw of many symptoms and complaints began to fit together. In 1971 in Dallas, I heard Mandell, Newbold, and Philpott give papers on cerebral allergy. After listening to these men, I came to the conclusion that these seemingly unexplainable symptoms in my patients could only be due to allergy. This was too much to accept all at once.

In 1974, I took the Roger J. Williams course in Rinkel allergy testing at Cheyenne, Wyoming. Ted Randolph was one of the speakers, and he reiterated his views of the previous year, with case reports to back him up. He told of fasting a patient for four days, then giving one food at a time. This would provoke the most outlandish symptomatology, but always something of which the patient had complained. Randolph could eliminate symptoms by fasting, then reproduce symptoms with foods and chemicals. He would even do this on demand! This was definitely allergy, and allergy would cause backache, headache, earache, or any other ache. Allergy could cause and did cause depression, mania, hyperactivity, or schizophrenia. Allergy could cause fatigue, lethargy, and hypoglycemia. This was to me a revelation, only because now I was ready to accept it at face value. The hypoglycemia diet had failed me and others. Vitamins had failed on some patients. Shock treatment never was too successful in this type of patient. Now I can understand why medical men have trouble accepting new concepts. Here I was, working in the field since 1968, refusing to believe Mandell in 1971, or Randolph in 1973. Only when the facts were demonstrated by personal experience did I permit myself to believe. It seems we all must learn the hard way.

By now, I was convinced of allergy as being the basic reason for many of the ills of man and took up Rinkel testing. Dr. Ivor Glaisher of Regina, Saskatchewan, showed me the practical side of the testing. I set up a lab with my wife in charge. In 1974, I spent a week with Dr. William H. Philpott. He was fasting and food testing, also using nutrients and many psychological techniques on his patients. In 1975, I visited Randolph's hospital for several days. All during this time, I was expanding the use of the four-day rotary, diversified diet, and nutrient therapy. I have fasted many patients using Randolph's technique and found his work to be factual, reproducible, and effective. By recognizing allergic symptoms as being due to allergens, whatever their nature, one is able to do much for patients. Best of all, one knows the cause of the patient's symptoms. A headache can be due to coffee, perfume, or a musty basement. Once a patient sees this relationship and, more important, is willing to correct it, he is well on the road to recovery.[63]

It is certainly unfortunate that all too often we scientists, physicians, and laymen must learn the hard way. Only with "the facts that are demonstrated by personal experience" do we permit ourselves to believe. In Green's case, he had to experience personally the symptomatic misery of low blood sugar before he began his quest for truth concerning this degenerative disease process. He, along with many others, began this quest with a corn-sugar test for hypoglycemia. The subsequent treatment was the traditional hypoglycemia diet (high protein, moderate fat, low carbohydrate) that was developed by Seale Harris, M.D., in 1924. This diet, he learned, worked "well for a time," but all too soon he began to experience what other physicians were telling him he would: that with this particular treatment, he would inflict upon himself new addiction to protein foods or to any other basic type of food that was frequently eaten and not rotated on at least a four-day basis. These newly established addictions would then radically alter his sugar levels and ultimately cause the reappearance of the very symptoms his previously poor diet of highly refined carbohydrate foods had initiated. Only by recognizing specific foods to which he was allergic, eliminating these foods for a few months, and then rotating them along with all his other foods, was Green able to feel good again.

It cannot be overemphasized that specific foods, whether protein, fat, or carbohydrate, as well as chemicals, can radically alter normal sugar levels into the states of hypo/hyperglycemia. No longer can we use the traditional corn-sugar test to determine that all carbohydrates should be reduced or eliminated from the diet. Any food or chemical that is frequently eaten or encountered has the potential of becoming addictive; and, as we have already discovered, any addictive substance can radically alter sugar levels. If your problems, therefore, were originally related to intake of carbohydrates, and you eliminate them in favor of eating a very high-protein diet—say, two to four eggs every day—it is very likely that within a few months or less those eggs, even though they are a superior food, loaded with many nutrients, and previously caused no symptoms, will make you feel very sick again. In order to avoid this type of symptomatic merry-go-round, the key points to remember are:

1. recognition of allergy specificity;
2. elimination of any incriminating substances from the diet or environment for two to four months; and
3. rotation of all foods, including previously addictive ones

The hard way to discover truth need not be the only one. We must always keep in mind that the greatest enemy of any science or any discovery of truth is a closed mind. Accordingly, we should continue to seek the courage to ask pertinent questions that will shake our complacency and challenge our minds to look deeper into the farthest reaches of the great mystery of the human body. Then and only then will we be able, as did Green, "to accept truth at face value."

Chapter 11

The Perils of Toximolecular Medicine: *Drug-Induced Illnesses*

Thus far we have been concerned with the roles played by nutritional deficiencies and allergic reactions in the initiation and progress of degenerative diseases. There is another class of illness that is peculiarly appalling because it is brought about by deliberate action, action undertaken with the best intention and with the sanction of medical authority, but nevertheless disastrous in its effects.

In my initial discussion of the orthomolecular approach to treatment, I touched on toximolecular medicine. This involves the administration of alien chemicals or drugs (substances not normally found in the human body) at sublethal levels in the treatment of infectious and degenerative diseases of all kinds. In mental and emotional illness, this includes giving patients a group of drugs known as phenothiazines and butyrophenones (referred to by the general term "neuroleptics") in dosages varying from very small to very large. Some examples of well-known antipsychotic drugs in this category are Stelazine, chlorpromazine, haloperidol, and fluphenazine. However, what is most interesting, and at the same time most tragic, about the neuroleptic drugs is the fact that when they are used over a period of time, which is often done in our psychiatric clinics for the mentally ill, the risk of evoking permanent injury to the liver, skin, cornea, bone marrow, heart, and especially to the central nervous system is greatly increased. Physicians as well as patients have a right to be alarmed at the growing list of evidences of adverse and even death-dealing reactions as a result of the chronic use of antipsychotic neuroleptic drugs. Consider, for instance, such side effects as allergic skin reactions, allergic bone marrow reactions producing agranulocytosis, liver destruction, hepatitis, as well as silent coronary death caused by drug-induced deterioration of the heart's conduction system. But probably the most well-known side effect of prolonged use of neuroleptic drugs is their tendency to produce a very serious central-nervous-system disorder known as tardive dyskinesia.

This condition is characterized by disturbed muscle movements, notably those of the face, and by tremor and rigidity in the hands and feet; memory and the ability to concentrate are also often drastically impaired. The dyskinetic finds himself involuntarily grimacing, chewing, sticking out his tongue, and blinking; he may also laugh or cry without feeling the emotions that would occasion these actions. Most of these patients live in a state of constant misery, isolated socially by their uncontrollable behavior and unable to perform any but the simplest tasks.

Past surveys[64] of chronically institutionalized population have reported the prevalence of tardive dyskinesia to range from 1 to 55 percent, with the most recent studies citing the highest percentages. These studies appeared to conclude that patients with high-risk levels of developing tardive dyskinesia were females, had been using neuroleptic medication for more than two years, and were older than fifty-five. Moreover, before a study done in 1977, it was commonly held that tardive dyskinesia was not a seriously prevalent problem among psychiatric outpatients being treated with neuroleptics, but rather was mainly a problem of chronically institutionalized patients. In 1977, this thinking changed. A group of physicians discovered to their dismay that 43.4 percent of a sample outpatient group had tardive dyskinesia. Previously, this group had been described as being "at nominal risk" of developing this dreadful disorder. What was even more disturbing about the results of this study was that the "dyskinetic group was relatively young (average age of 45.5 years), had a short duration of neuroleptic medication (less than two years), and were not chronically hospitalized."[65] The study also reported that "there was no significant relationship between the presence of dyskinesia and age, sex, years of neuroleptic use, history of electric shock treatment, amphetamine or alcohol abuse, or of neurological disorders in the patients or their families."[66] The researchers concluded that outpatients, as well as institutionalized patients, receiving neuroleptics were being given a form of treatment that substantially raised the patient's risk of developing tardive dyskinesia.

Due to the seriousness and widespread occurrence of tardive dyskinesia, the Food and Drug Administration (FDA) as far back as 1973 recommended that physicians minimize the use of neuroleptics in chronically ill patients and especially in those patients over the age of fifty.[67] The FDA also suggested that many patients could be maintained for long periods of time without antipsychotic drugs. The agency's bulletin further advised that neuroleptics should be immediately discontinued whenever any signs, symptoms, or manifestations of tardive dyskinesia appeared; it has been documented that these initial symptoms may be irreversible.

The one tragic aspect of tardive dyskinesia is that it is often not responsive to treatment with the usual drug arsenal of anticholinergic or antiparkinson agents. "The occurrence of immediate extrapyramidal symptoms due to treatment with neuroleptics," writes Richard Kunin, M.D., "is so commonplace that it has become routine to prescribe anticholinergic-type antiparkinson agents along with the antipsychotic drugs. Antiparkinson drugs, such as benztropine mesylate (Cogentin®), trihexyphenidyl (Artane®), or procyclidine (Kemadrin®) usually attenuate the immediate extrapyramidal symptoms, but they definitely increase the risk of tardive dyskinesia. In addition, they sometimes interfere with treatment of psychosis by aggravating hostility reactions, and in some cases they cause a toxic, confusional state."[68]

The physician faced with the problem of treating tardive dyskinesia by conventional methods has few choices, none of them appealing. He may decrease the dosage of the neuroleptic drug, aware that the condition has been induced by the drug; but the damage has already been done. He may increase the dosage in order to suppress the symptoms, but any good effect will be only temporary; and the same, as Dr. Kunin indicates, is true of the use of anticholinergic antiparkinson agents.

Far too often, the grotesque movements symptomatic of the disorder are interpreted by medical and nursing personnel as manifestations of madness or hysteria, to be attacked by the use of drugs to "suppress the nervousness" or psychotherapy to "get at the underlying conflicts." Thus the patient is seen as the source of the problem—which actually is a result of the initial decision to employ toximolecular medicine. There are few better examples of what is called iatrogenic (physician-induced) illness.

We have seen that the orthomolecular approach to treatment has resulted in startling benefits in cases of disease that have defied treatment by other means. Research has now begun to show the possibility of similar results with tardive dyskinesia, with evidence of the destructive effects of neuroleptic drugs on mineral and vitamin levels in the body and the consequently indicated course of attacking the disease by rectifying these nutrient levels.

Dr. Kunin was one of the first researchers to discover the relationship between these drugs and depleted nutrient levels. Let us examine some of the personal case histories that gave him new insights into an effective form of treatment for tardive dyskinesia.

> With the earlier of these cases, having tried antiparkinson agents and rauwolfia to no avail, I recalled that phenothiazines are potent chelators of manganese. I also recalled that manganese is found in high concentration in the extrapyramidal system. I reasoned that phenothiazines might chelate manganese, thus binding it electrochemically, and that this might make manganese unavailable for some presumed function as an enzyme activator. It seemed plausi-

ble that by providing extra dietary manganese the deficiency would be corrected and the dyskinesia might thereby improve.

I did not have long to wait before a young man (see case five in Table 11.1) consulted me because of dyskinesia due to fluphenazine enanthate (Prolixin®). This had been administered over two months earlier at a university psychiatric service in two doses of 100 milligrams, intramuscularly, a week apart, plus 30 milligrams orally for four days and 45 milligrams for four more days. He still exhibited masklike facial expression, Parkinson's posture and gait, and severe tremor and rigidity of the extremeties. These symptoms had persisted in spite of previous treatment with diphenhydramine (Benedryl®), diazepam (Valium®), and nicotinamide (1,000 milligrams, t.i.d.). Manganese chelate, 10 milligrams, t.i.d., was now started. After one day, the tremor and rigidity were much improved. After two days, he was entirely free of dyskinesia. There was no recurrence.

Another young man (see case seven in Table 11.1) was treated with fluphenazine (Prolixin), 30 milligrams per day, orally for ten months in a state hospital for his second schizophrenic episode. During his previous hospitalization of six months' duration, four years earlier, he was treated with chlorpromazine, 150 milligrams, t.i.d. In each illness, he had taken LSD beforehand. He had terminated fluphenazine and trihexyphenidyl (Artane) nine weeks earlier, but still had parkinsonian posture, masklike face, and moderate tremor of the thumb and forefinger. On a low dose of manganese chelate, 6.4 milligrams per day, in a multivitamin, he showed no improvement in two weeks. However, when the dose was increased by the addition of manganese chelate, 5 milligrams, t.i.d., providing a total of 21.4 milligrams of manganese per day, he showed overnight improvement in posture and gait and more gradual improvement in facial expression. Mental dullness and flat affect did not improve until he was treated with nicotinic acid (vitamin B_3), 250 milligrams, t.i.d., three months later.[69]

Table 11.1 summarizes Kunin's observations of fifteen cases of manganese therapy for tardive dyskinesia. The tabulation shows that in fifteen cases of tardive dyskinesia treated with manganese,

TABLE 11.1. *Dr. Kunin's Observations of Fifteen Cases of Manganese Therapy for Tardive Dyskinesia*

Case #	Diagnosis	Age Sex	Drug	Duration Avg. Dose	Dyskinesia	Mn Hair	Result/Mn	Result/B_3
1.	Neurotic	61	Thiordazine	1½ yr.	Oral, Buccal	0.2	Much improved	Improved
	Depression	Male			Glossal		Cured	
					Akathisia		Much improved	
2.	Paranoid	46	Chlorpromazine	15 yr.	Eyelid Closure	0.6	Improved	
	Schizophrenia	Male		200 mg/d	Akathisia		Improved	
					Oral		Improved	
			Haloperidol	2 yr.				
				10 mg/d				
3.	Neurotic	70	Thioridazine	11 yr.	Tremor	0.4	Improved	
	Depression	Fem.		150 mg/d	(arms)			
4.	Anxiety	25	Thioridazine	5 yr.	Glossal	0.4	Cured	
	Disorder	Male		75 mg/d	Cervical		Cured	
5.	Paranoid	20	Fluphenazine	12 days	Tremor	1.0	Cured	
	Schizophrenia	Male		45 mg/d	Rigidity		Cured	
				100 mg IMx2				
6.	Schizoaffective	39	Chlorpromazine	16 yr.	Tremor	0.6	Improved	Much improved
		Fem.		400 mg/d	Akathisia		Improved	Much improved
					Oral		Unchanged	Unchanged
			Haloperidol	1½ yr.	Tremor		Improved	Improved
				1 mg				
7.	Paranoid	23	Fluphenazine	1½ yr.	Rigidity	0.3	Cured	
	Schizophrenic	Male		30 mg/d	Tremor		Cured	
			Chlorpromazine	600 mg				

8.	Schizoaffective	28 Male	Chlorpromazine Haloperidol Thiothixene	7 yr. 200 mg/d 7 days 20 mg/d 3 mos. 15 mg/d	Akathisia	0.3	Cured	
9.	Schizoaffective	25 Male	Fluphenazine	7 yr. 20 mg/d	Tremor Rigidity Akathisia	0.6	Cured Cured Cured	
10.	Paranoid Schizophrenic	18 Male	Fluphenazine Mesondazine Thiothixene	½ yr. 75 mg/wk ½ yr. 150 mg/d ½ yr. 40 mg/d	Tremor Rigidity	0.2	Unchanged Unchanged	Cured Cured
11.	Manic Depressive	50 Male	Fluphenazine	10 yr. 10 mg/d	Tremor	0.6	Cured	
12.	Paranoid Schizophrenia	22 Male	Fluphenazine Trifluoperazine	3 mos. 25 mg/wk 2 yrs. 20 mg/d	Tremor Rigidity Akathisia	0.3	 Much improved Improved	
13.	Schizophrenia (Undiff.)	30 Fem.	Fluphenazine Haloperidol	½ yr. 125 mg/wk ½ yr. 110 mg/d	Oculogyric	0.7	Cured	Much improved
14.	Schizoaffective	36 Fem.	Trifluoperazine	9 yr. 5 mg/d	Tremor Akathisia	0.6	Cured Improved	
15.	Paranoid Schizophrenia	38 Fem.	Trifluoperazine	6 yr. 8 mg/d	Oral Akathisia	0.2	Much improved	

seven (46 percent) were cured outright (cases 4, 5, 7, 8, 9, 11, 13). Three (20 percent) cases were much improved (cases 1, 6, 12). Four (27 percent) were improved (cases 2, 3, 14, 15), and only one (7.7 percent) was unimproved after treatment with manganese (case 10). Moreover, according to Kunin, not included in the tabulation were his observations, which indicated that those cases that showed prompt response to manganese also showed complete response: that is, there were four cases (cases 5, 8, 11, 13) of literally overnight, complete cures. In nine other cases, a definite improvement was noticed in two to five days. Also of interest is the fact that all of the dramatic results were in patients age fifty or under.

Case 10 did not respond to manganese therapy but did dramatically get better upon introducing vitamin B_3. Dr. Kunin describes this case in more detail.

> The patient was an eighteen-year-old schizophrenic college student whose dyskinesia appeared while he was under treatment for six months with fluphenazine, mesoridazine, and thiothixene. The dyskinesia erupted full force with sever tremor of the extremities and severe rigidity. Manganese was of no benefit at a dose of up to 80 milligrams per day. Then, after ten weeks without improvement, there was complete and sustained relief within three hours of a single, oral dose of niacin (vitamin B_3), 500 milligrams. The niacin flush reaction frightened the patient so that he delayed three days before taking a second dose. During this time, the dyskinesia partially recurred. The second dose of niacin produced a complete cure.[70]

Dr. Kunin reports that vitamin B_3 at dosages of 100 to 500 milligrams was of significant benefit in treating the dyskinesia in three of the fifteen listed cases (cases 1, 10, 13). In another case (case 7), niacin "improved mental acuity," but it was not given until after the manganese treatment for the tardive dyskinesia had already been successful.

In order to give credence to the idea that phenothiazines chelate and thus remove manganese from the body by sequestering the ion in an electrochemical bond, Kunin ran spectrographic mineral hair analyses on a number of dyskinesia patients as well as nondyskinesia patients. He discovered that the nondyskinesia patients had an average of 0.8 parts per million of manganese in their hair. The dyskinesia group had only 0.46 parts per million, which was nearly 50 percent less than the control group. This evidence would suggest that neuroleptic treatment may induce a manganese deficiency in susceptible or borderline deficient patients.

Two other recent scientific studies give evidence that specific nutrients can help in the treatment of tardive dyskinesia. John H. Growdon, M.D., headed a team of researchers who gave pharmacologic doses of the nutrient choline to patients with stable tardive dyskinesia. Their goal was to suppress all involuntary facial movements in these patients. Choline is a physiologic precursor of acetylcholine, and its administration elevates brain acetylcholine levels in laboratory animals; it is hypothesized that choline will do the same in human beings. The researchers thought it could help tardive dyskinesia patients because, they maintained, the disorder is a result of a "deficiency of central cholinergic tone."[71] Twenty patients with tardive dyskinesia took oral doses of choline for two weeks in accordance with double-blind scientific protocol. Facial movements decreased significantly in nine of the patients, worsened in one, and were unchanged in the remaining ten. The study concluded that "oral doses of choline can be useful in neurologic diseases in which an increase in acetylcholine release is desired."

The second scientific study worked with five tardive-dyskinesia patients. These patients manifested orofacial dyskinesia, which first appeared after the discontinuation of neuroleptic drugs. They were observed for a minimum of two months to ensure that the movement disorder was stable prior to testing. One thousand to fourteen hundred milligrams of vitamin B_6 were tested on these patients. Joe DeVeaugh-Geiss, M.D., concluded that "four of the five patients showed a reduction in frequency of involuntary movements while on pyridoxine, which was sustained as long as B_6 was administered. . . . Pyridoxine appears to have a favorable effect on the movement disorder of tardive dyskinesia."[72]

The implications of these three studies on manganese, niacin, choline, and B_6 are far-reaching. Since the use of neuroleptic drugs appears to cause a deficiency of these nutrients, the question arises as to what other nutrient deficiencies might occur as a result of chronic tranquilizer use. What about amino acids, other vitamins, minerals, trace elements, and enzymes, all of which might be adversely affected by continual neuroleptic drug therapy? If neuroleptic drugs have the power to chelate manganese out of the body, they certainly have the potential of occasioning other nutritional deficiencies not yet recognized by physicians who continue their search for a new "wonder drug" while their patients' bodies and brain chemistries are crying out for chemicals (nutrients) that have existed in the human body since the beginning of time.

If there is one thing that our study of tardive dyskinesia can teach us, it is that we can no longer be content to search for some new drug that will help cure the ill effects of already existing drugs. Rather, we must begin looking to the human body and, more specifically, to each cell of the body as a teacher of medical wisdom. For it is in a total understanding of the complex function of the cell and the forty-plus nutrients needed by each cell for optimum health and life that physicians and scientists will be able to win the battle now waged against mental illness in specific and degenerative disease in general. In addition to this, we must also redirect our attention to the environmental factors (i.e., chemicals, foods, infections), which can precipitate symptoms of illness in patients. In short, orthomolecular nutrient therapy, which shifts the vital biochemical balance toward a more healthy response to stress by strengthening enzyme, immunological, hormonal, and other internal nutritionally based systems, coupled with ecologic environmental control, which seeks to identify and control all incompatible, stress-inducing environmental exposures, will ultimately prove to be the medical approach that truly meets the patient's biochemical and psychological needs at all levels.

In years to come, it will very likely be demonstrated that the most serious consequence of tranquilization is the speeding up of the diabetes mellitus disease process. Reports already reveal a four- to fivefold increase in maturity-onset diabetes in tranquilized patients compared to nontranquilized. This fact involves all types of tranquilizers, minor as well as major. Diabetes carries with it an array of complications affecting multiple organ systems, early development of artherosclerosis, reduced resistance to infection, and in some cases premature death. This is understandable in terms of ours and others' findings that maturity-onset diabetes is the logical end product of the stress of prolonged addiction to foods, chemicals, and inhalants. The mechanism is that these addicted patients are already in the prediabetic (chemical diabetic) phase, and when additionally addicted to tranquilizers they are further rapidly advanced to the chemical phase of maturity-onset diabetes.

Indeed, two state hospitals (Camarillo State Hospital in California and Central State Hospital in Oklahoma) have undergone court hearings because of the increased death rates in these institutions. Their defense was realistic: Our doctors are not negligent, but our patients are tranquilized, which creates two problems.

1. The muscles used for swallowing are affected; sometimes when they try to swallow they inhale instead, which draws food and mucus into their lungs by mistake.
2. The tranquilizers have also reduced their resistance to infection.

Our tranquilized patients are dying of lung infections they cannot immunologically handle. The lowered resistance to infection is typical of the advancing of the diabetes mellitus disease process.

This candid admission from the practitioners of present-day, toximolecular psychiatry is important to an understanding of both the doctor's and patient's plight when tranquilizers are used. Surely doctors and patients alike have a right to an alternative to the obviously damaging treatment of tranquilization.

Chapter 12

Angela's Chance at Life: *Autism Unraveled*

There are over ten million hyperactive or autistic children in the United States today. With these numbers increasing daily, it is important for us to understand that orthomolecular-ecologic medicine can help these children to create for themselves more healthy, creative, and meaningful lives. The following case history of an autistic child, as told by the mother and confirmed by the referring psychologist, is given as evidence of this fact. If the future of our nation lies in the hearts and minds of our children, our hope for a more creative society will certainly be brightened by little Angela's story of personal struggle, treatment, and continuing development and success in spite of her inherited biochemical limitations.

Angela's Case History

February 26, 1976[73]

It's hard to believe Angela is the same little girl as six months ago. Her gentleness and sensitivity is reblossoming. She is becoming her own person. I watch with a mother's joy how my four-year-old daughter is exploring her world for the first time. And best of all, her affection is growing for those around her. It wasn't so long ago Angela was a hyperactive, whining, tantrum-throwing, confused child that was locked in a world alone; unreachable.

Angela had been a healthy baby physically. Our doctor would jot down "everything perfect" on her health book after each checkup. He said she was doing fine and had nothing to worry about. And if I felt a little apprehensive, it was just new-mother blues and would pass. Her crying spells were probably from being immunized, a touch of colic, or even an allergy to the flowers that everyone sent me when she was born. She'll settle down, he reassured me. I was just tired from my new duties as first-time mother, and this caused needless concern over my new baby. But with each passing week, the doctor's words of comfort were lost in the almost constant, inconsolable wailing of my daughter.

I began to notice that Angela became overly agitated and upset when there were too many people around her. The first time I was sure of this was at her christening. She was a month old. Angela screamed throughout the ceremony and was upset for most of the day. It had turned into an ordeal for both of us, and I was worn out with nervous exhaustion by that night. Angela wasn't much better. Nothing seemed to comfort her except my mother-in-law rocking her. She would doze off, but as soon as Grandma would stop rocking to get up, Angela would wake with a start and begin to cry again. There were many sleepless nights before and after that. My husband and I took turns rocking her at all hours. It was the only thing that seemed to calm her.

I had a feeling something was very wrong with Angela, only I couldn't put my finger on it. I felt helpless, and I worried. When I took her in for her checkups, I just didn't know how to explain my feelings to the doctor. Later, when Angela was three years old, he told me she seemed unhappy. That's all he could tell me, because physically she was perfect.

Angela had not learned any words by her first birthday, not even "mama." She seemed to be developing her motor skills normally, but socially she seemed detached and hardly smiled. She was content to be left behind by her father and me when we went out. She rarely even noticed our presence when we would try to get her attention. My husband and his parents refused to believe anything was wrong. "She'll grow out of it," they told me. It was tearing me apart inside. My baby didn't even know me as her mother. I was a stranger and an intruder into her growing isolation.

Angela's second year was worse than her first. She began throwing tantrums, screaming loudly, and kicking for no apparent reason.

I had become pregnant with our second child, and I thought this might have had something to do with it. She began spending hours in her open closet, picking up little toys and watching them drop over and over. Or she would lie in her crib and stare at the ceiling or walls for long periods. If I called her name, she made no movement to come; she didn't even look up at me. If I interfered with what she was doing by picking her up, she would just stiffen and scream. It was as though she preferred objects to people.

Angela also became afraid of things. A crack in a wall or a corner in a ceiling would just terrify her. She would run out of the room in hysterics, just to abruptly turn and stare wide-eyed and shaking at the spot on the wall that had frightened her so. She reacted the same way to the sounds of vacuum cleaners, blenders, sewing machines, or lawnmowers. Shaking with fear, she would scream until I turned them off. Some nights I would awaken to her shrieking. I would pick her up and rock her until she was calm enough to lie down again. Then I would lie next to her and hum softly until one of us fell asleep.

When Angela was eighteen months old, Diego, our son, was born. The birth had gone exceptionally well in spite of my growing anxiety over Angela. She had spent the last days of my pregnancy with her grandma. The first night she came home, she came into the bedroom and crawled up on the bed where Diego and I were. She was upset and it sounded like she said, "Baby, baby, baby!" That night, Diego, Angela, and I slept together. It would be the only social gesture of needing me that she would make for some time to come.

Angela's second birthday came and went with no improvement. She still used no words. Her strange behavior took on new dimensions. When I would pick her up, she would go limp rather than hold on; she avoided looking at us. She seemed lost in a world of her own. Friends and relatives who came over would make up to Diego, but they would tend to overlook Angela. Her father even began to leave her to herself. I found it easier to let her play undisturbed. So it went. We were losing our daughter to an invisible world.

Angela's antisocial behavior did not escape our friends' notice either. One person suggested she might be tongue-tied. The doctor said no. Another friend said maybe she had trouble hearing. We took her to a speech and hearing clinic. They tested her and said she could hear. Our search for answers was endless.

Meanwhile, Diego was growing. His eyes would follow Angela everywhere. I remember one day Angela got too close, so he reached out and firmly grabbed her by the hair. I had to pry his little fingers loose. He chuckled at what he had done. He was thoroughly fascinated by her. She, likewise, began to show curiosity in him. At six months old, Diego was crawling after her and loved watching her play with toys. Usually it was the toy she had just taken away from him. I began to realize there was a special relationship developing between them, and it gave me hope for Angela.

At three years old, Angela was still totally nonverbal. She could not tell us of her needs, where she hurt, or anything. In spite of Angela's being antisocial, though, Diego was not allowing her to stay in her isolated world. Rejection didn't bother him. As soon as he could walk, he would grab her or chase after her. He would take toys from her and she was forced to respond. She would look right at him and yell in anger or give him a good push. He thought the whole thing was comical, unless she got too rough with him. I watched how my son, only a year and a half old, had opened up a line of communication with Angela. There was a growing trust and affection between them. Many times Angela would look at him or touch him, something she had never done with us. Diego had entered her world. She acknowledged and accepted his presence in her room while other children were outsiders that she would move away from or scream at if cornered. I decided to do what my small son had done: break the wall down. The key was persistence and simple faith. Time was running short for Angela and soon she would be facing school.

The task of changing everybody's habits toward Angela was not so easy. Her father and I argued about it. I know Angela's rejecting and ignoring him hurt very much. But I convinced him to make the effort. He would pick her up to say hello and make a fuss over her regularly whether she liked it or not. She slowly began to respond to the attention everyone was suddenly paying her. I would sit and hold her on my lap and play pat-a-cake or sing nursery rhymes even if she didn't seem to pay attention. When people came in, I would remind them to say hello to Angela, too, and make a fuss over her as well as Diego. Even though she still did not look at us, she no longer squirmed to get down when we picked her up. She even began to come into the living room when someone came over. I began to realize how important our attitude was as an example to other people. How we treated Angela was how they would treat her.

It was about a month after Angela turned three that I happened to see a TV program on autistic children. The past three years of unanswered questions suddenly came into sharp focus. I never dreamed Angela's strange behavior was a rare brain disorder affecting an average of four in ten thousand children.

Not long after that, a relative gave me a newspaper article on a project at UCLA involving autistic children. I called to make an appointment. I wanted a doctor who worked with autistic children to confirm or deny my fears. It was true: Angela was autistic. When the doctor told us after observing her, it didn't make us feel any better or worse. Only now, Angela's problem had an official name.

That fall, I went to the local college and took nursery school education classes. My mother-in-law was kind enough to watch the children. What I learned that semester has helped me understand what all children need, regardless of handicap.

The following semester I decided to enroll Angela in the college's day-care center. I thought being with other children might help her socially. They accepted her at the center on a trial basis because I told them she was autistic. At first everything went well. Angela seemed happy to go. It was about a month later that Angela's teacher began to hint that it was not working out with Angela. The pressure and tension began to mount with each passing day. Comments, advice, criticism, and finally incredible accusations from my daughter's teacher forced me to withdraw her from the center. It was then that I learned the painful truth: that the other parents had filed complaints, not wanting their children around Angela; and that my own teachers at the college had been at a staff meeting to decide how to handle the problem. I solved their "problem" by taking my child back home. After such an experience, I had no desire to finish school.

But everything has a purpose, and one teacher gave me a brochure on the 1975 National Autistic Conference to be held in San Diego. My husband was enthusiastic about going. What better place to find out every alternative open to us for Angela?

The conference lasted four days. In that time, a new world opened up to us. We listened to lectures, heard the stories other parents had to tell of their autistic children, and talked to doctors from different fields about their theories on the subject. One presentation in particular impressed us. It was on allergies that affect the brain and central nervous system and megavitamin therapy. I had suspected some foods were affecting Angela adversely. Here were professionals who thought the same way. We got the name of a medical doctor in our area who specialized in neurological allergies. When we came home, we set up an appointment to meet him.

Soon after that, Angela, her father, and I went to Dana Point where Dr. Philpott had his clinic. I was a little nervous with anticipation as we waited. Angela was irritable. She never liked waiting. Her father was quiet. When we were ushered into his office, Angela would not sit still. She ran in and out of the room, at times pausing to rock back and forth and giggle, turning the light switch off and on as it caught her fancy. She was oblivious to anyone in the room. In spite of the interruptions, Dr. Philpott presented us with his reasons for feeling he could help us. He had a complete routine worked out for testing patients with mild to severe "unexplainable" mental, emotional, or physical disorders, from an ecological standpoint, that is, what was affecting them adversely in their daily lives in the way of food, chemicals, and other environmental factors. In this way, he tracked down and weeded out substances causing a reaction, whether mental, emotional, or physical. Then an individual four-day rotation diet was worked out with foods that didn't have a reaction. What he said made a lot of sense to us. We put Angela under his care.

In the five weeks that followed, my daughter and I became closer than I ever thought possible. Every day for five weeks (except Saturday and Sunday), Angela and I would leave early in the morning for the clinic. We would stay until late afternoon. Angela was given three test meals a day. Each meal was one particular food. Blood sugar was monitored along with pulse and urine within two hours after each meal. Changes in behavior, mood, color of face, or anything else observed that indicated a reaction was noted in diary form. I was shown how to take a pulse, as it needed to be taken every fifteen minutes during the test. We ended up using a stethoscope for Angela since she wouldn't stand still long enough for me to find her pulse.

Some days she had terrible reactions, especially in the first two weeks. She would be peaceful before eating wheat, for instance, but within fifteen minutes after ingesting it, the color drained from her face, she broke out in a sweat, and with eyes half-closed she went into a stupor. She had the same reaction to oats, only more severe and longer lasting, ending up with her sleeping it off in the afternoon. I was amazed. Equally astounding was what fruit did to her blood sugar. One hundred and sixty milligrams percent is top normal after a meal. At one hour after these test meals, Angela had 400 for apples, 240 for mangos, 300 for watermelon, 240 for cantaloupe, 300 for oranges, 400 for pineapple, 400 for grapes, 400 for apricots, and 320 for blueberries. She became very hyperactive, too. Foods I thought so wholesome and good were incriminated.

By the end of three weeks, Angela had begun to connect sitting on her potty chair with urinating so she began to hold it until I put her on. That was a miracle in itself. The fifth week was devoted to chemical sublingual drop tests. Food coloring, especially red, sent her into a stupor. Insecticides were also reactive. The test for hydrocarbon reaction made her go pale, break out in a sweat, and become extremely irritable.

By the end of the fifth week, Angela had panties on instead of a diaper, and she began to go on the toilet. No one could have convinced me Angela would be toilet-trained five weeks before. And the five weeks we spent together during the ups and downs of the testing really made me feel like Angela's mother in a special way. She needed me and came to me for comfort for the first time. She understood when I asked her if she wanted to go home by taking my hand. She began to recognize our car in the parking lot. Most of all, she had become so much calmer and happier in those five weeks. Her father and his whole family were very impressed by the change in Angela. Not half as much as I, though.

We had much to thank Dr. Philpott and his wife for. Without their pioneering spirit and independent thinking, Angela would not be the carefree, happy child that enjoys living now. Instead, she would still be a very sick little girl, and we would be a helpless, frustrated family. I'm not saying this in flattery, but in absolute truth.

And what has happened to Angela since the test? She became fully potty-trained three months later. She began to notice things in the house and explored as if she had been blind and could suddenly see. Each day has brought new, subtle changes in Angela. It's as if she is slowly waking from a deep sleep. For the first time, she is taking interest in what people are doing around her. Her eye contact with her family is good, and it is improving with outsiders. She plays with toys more appropriately now, and she has lost much of her repetitive mannerisms. Just lately, she has become very attached to me and will not let me out the front door, or let me take a shower, or let me leave the room without her following me. A two-year-old child goes through such a phase. Angela never went through it. She's got a lot of catching up to do. She no longer wants to be left behind. She will come into whatever room we happen to be sitting in and climb up into her dad's lap to watch TV; or she'll pull me to sit down with her while she looks through a book; or she'll just come and sit in close proximity to wherever we happen to be. For the first time we really feel like a family and it's wonderful. All of these things may sound trivial to someone who has never experienced an autistic child, but, believe me, it is something to celebrate for us!

After attending a week-long diagnostic session for Angela, she started school a little over a month ago and is doing fine. This time it is a special-education class at a local public grammar school. They are using sign language as an intermediate step to speech, successfully with Angela. I am very impressed with the methods and the staff. They show much compassion and understanding of an autistic child's needs and problems. I plan on writing my state officials to that effect.

Life is no longer treading water for Angela. She is swimming for home. With the continued diet Dr. Philpott devised for her, meganutrients, going to school, and a whole lot of love and patience from those around her, I know Angela will have a chance at life.

Donna M. Calvera (Angela's mother)

Mother's Progress Report October 11, 1976

Angela began talking about a year after she went through the initial four-day fast for Dr. Philpott's food allergy testing (July 1975). I believe there were presteps to her verbalizing.

1. Angela's receptive language accelerated geometrically within a month after being on the rotation diet. Potty training was an immediate by-product. By January 1976, she understood not just words but could carry out simple verbal directions, such as "sit down", "go to bed", "stand up", "time to eat", and "take a bath". By the beginning of March 1976, Angela was carrying out more complicated instructions, such as "take this to your room", "put these pants on", "put your toys away", and "take your clothes off". In June 1976, Angela stayed with her grandma for three weeks and was following instructions in Spanish without difficulty. This was without the strict use of behavior modification. It seemed to come naturally (although at her school they use positive reinforcement only).
2. In January 1976, Angela began a public school special-education class here in Whittier that uses positive reinforcement only in the area of behavior modification. The program utilizes sign language as an intermediate step to verbal communication. Within the first two weeks, Angela understood her teachers' basic signs to her. They motored her through the basic signs and in April she was spontaneously using those signs to communicate her needs, such as eat, potty, and play.
3. This initial breakthrough in communication for Angela gave her a whole new awareness about her world. She now wanted to be

understood by others; she made the effort to be understood. Her using the sign for eating got her immediate results, which delighted her. With each sign came much approval and affection from those around her (especially me!). She was aware that she was causing a good kind of excitement by signing, which gave her obvious pleasure.

4. Acquiring one sign after another seemed to accelerate and made it easier for Angela to imitate those around her, not just in signing, but in many other activities, such as play and helping.
5. By the end of May 1976, Angela was picking up signs as fast as any normal child would and retaining them, which is another crucial difference in her since she's been on the diet. I would make a completely new sign and after showing her two times, she would imitate me. (She is on the level of learning naming signs and has not gone into more abstract communication.)
6. Angela's retaining the signs, learning them so fast, and using them so spontaneously gave me the wherewithal to push her to verbalize her needs one night. It was an incredibly simple step for her to imitate my sound of "mama." I repeated it three times, elaborating. She got the idea and attempted to imitate my sound. It was the first clear-cut imitation of language I ever witnessed from Angela. She looked me straight in the eye when she said it, and I almost wept for joy! I got her to say it again and again; she thought it was a game and giggled, enjoying my excitement. That initial verbal breakthrough spawned a whole series of imitative sounds. Her first phrase was "eat food," pronounced "ee! oo!" and, believe me, she knew what she was saying!
7. It's been about two months now since her first "mama" and "eat food." We've added "go home," "bye-bye," "hi," "I want ———," "get drink," "take bath," "go play," and a lot of others. Actually, she'll make an attempt at imitating any word I ask her to. Longer words confuse her though. She goes through the ABCs and 1-2-3s with me; also everyone's name, the parts of the body, and the like. She really enjoys these communication games. (The idea for this came from *Sesame Street* on TV, which she watches now.)
8. At this point, I feel Angela's receptive language is 100 percent, spontaneous speech is 30 percent (being high incentive), imita-

tive or cued speech is 80 to 85 percent. Angela's retention, memory, and verbal imitation are very high. Her comprehension falls within the limits of immediate personal needs and naming objects.

Angela enjoys verbalizing and realizes that a magic barrier that separated her from other people has disappeared, which has helped her surge forward in spontaneous social contact. She is very affectionate and is learning social behavior without being prodded into it.

Finally, I must repeat in all sincerity that there has been an about-face in Angela in every respect since going on her allergy-free diet. The list is long of all the dramatic changes that have taken place over this past year, from potty training to talking. We couldn't ask for more as a family.

My fond hope is that food and chemical testing—clinical ecology—can someday be used in the processing and screening of developmentally disabled children and adults to at least rule out the possibility of allergy-caused disorders.

Angela was a confirmed case of autism—childhood psychosis—by Dr. Ivar Lovass and Dr. Simmons of UCLA in 1974. She was a completely incoherent, hyperactive mess then. We went another year with no help and no progress in Angela. Dr. Philpott took her on as a patient in July 1975. Now, one year later, Angela is a different child, as if she was never that bad and all the heartache was a collective nightmare for our family.

Comment by Bernard Rimland, Ph.D., October 14, 1976

I am very proud to have had a hand in the near-miraculous improvement of Angela Calvera. I met Angela's parents at the 1975 convention of the National Society for Autistic Children in San Diego. They told me about Angela, and when I discovered that they lived within a short distance of Dr. Philpott's office, I urged that they take Angela to him. It was not long before I began receiving a series of excited telephone calls and letters from Mrs. Calvera, who could hardly believe the improvement that was taking place before her eyes.

In May of 1976, I had my first opportunity to meet Angela. I was speaking at a conference on autism near the Calvera's residence, and Mrs. Calvera brought Angela to me during one of the intermissions. Angela was a beautiful and well-behaved little girl. After the intermission, I began talking about my scheduled topic, "Nutrition As It Relates to Autism and Other Severe Learning Disorders." With Mrs. Calvera's permission, I mentioned the case to the audience; then I invited Mrs. Calvera and Angela to come to the podium. Mrs. Calvera spoke briefly about her experience and the marvelous improvement that had taken place in Angela. But interested as the audience was in Mrs. Calvera's talk, all eyes were actually riveted to Angela, who was sitting at the speaker's table, confronted with several long-stemmed and very fragile-looking water glasses. Angela picked one up very carefully, sipped a little water, and placed it down on the table very carefully. You couldn't have asked to see a more normal-appearing and well-behaved child. Angela demonstrated to that audience of several hundred people much more eloquently than I could have that the methods of clinical ecology, as embodied in the work of Dr. Philpott and his colleagues, are indeed effective and can often bring about behavioral improvements which border on the incredible.

Discussion

We need all the help we can get from diagnostic or treatment modalities for learning-disabled, hyperkinetic, autistic, and psychotic children. No one in any discipline has anything more than partial answers, and we desperately need all the answers we can get. I submit that an ecologic examination of these problems reveals clinical ecology to be one of these partial answers. Even when there is a demonstrated evidence of symptom production on exposure to a food or chemical, we still do not know why. Are the varied reasons for reactions immunological, metabolic errors, enzyme deficiencies, nutritional deficiencies, toxins, infections, or something else? It could be any or all of these. Only years of detailed research will tell us some of these facts.

Angela has not been cured by avoiding symptom-incriminated foods and taking nutritional supplements that correspond to her demonstrated nutritional needs. She will have to lead a carefully regulated life of food rotation, avoidance of certain chemicals, and supernutrition supplements as long as she lives. Successful living for her will always be a matter of maintaining a precarious metabolic balance. It is hoped that in the future, research will have defined the deficient enzymes, which can then be supplemented and thus provide for her a less regimented life.

One thing stands out in her case, as it has in all such cases I have examined, and that is the provocative test evoking of a disordered carbohydrate metabolism of hyperglycemia. These findings of disordered carbohydrate metabolism are consistent with the prediabetic state termed chemical diabetes mellitus. I have observed that the chemistry of any addictive state, whether to foods or chemicals, is a carbohydrate disorder that can be evoked by fats, proteins, and nonfood inhalants to which the subject is symptom reactive as well as to only selective carbohydrates.

Angela is most fortunate to have parents who care, and who have intelligently proceeded with the necessary educational and psychotherapeutic pursuits without which she still would fail to mature psychologically.

AFTERWORD

The authors of this book, unlike most medical writers, include in their purview the facts of inborn biochemical individuality and the additional fact that the numerous nutrients are typically not like medicines picking away at specific diseases, but they work together as a team to promote healthy metabolism.

Now that it is clear from the work of E. Arthur Robertson, Andre C. Van Steirteghem, James E. Byrkit, and Donald S. Young, published in *Clinical Chemistry*, that everyone has a metabolic pattern all his or her own, it becomes more obvious that disease may occur in selected individuals simply because they have genetic nutrient needs that are difficult to meet.[74] Likewise, genetically derived individuality causes people to react very differently to potentially deleterious substances. Degenerative diseases and mental troubles are indeed complex and ramifications may occur.

The importance of our internal environments, consisting not only of at least forty essential nutrients—minerals, trace minerals, amino acids, and vitamins—but also an unknown number of substances that can be harmful, would be difficult to exaggerate. Attempts to solve individual health problems often require careful detective work and at this stage of our development success cannot be guaranteed. However, we have many more clues to follow now than we had a decade ago.

Without an appreciation of the importance of this internal environment—how nutrition works and how adverse elements can creep in and interfere with metabolism—the solution to many individual health problems is hopeless.

Since the writers of this book are aware of these concepts, they have written a volume that presents, in a highly important way, a modern outlook.

—ROGER J. WILLIAMS, PH.D.

APPENDIX FOR PHYSICIANS

My hoped-for audience thus far for this book has been twofold. For the lay reader, I have presented as well as I could the evidence for a new view of the many specific conditions and of the nature of the basic disease process. Aside from following certain basic rules on nutrition and supplementation, and being alert for signs of the presence of an allergic-addictive reaction, there is little that can be done on one's own. However, it is important that everyone be informed as fully as possible on so vital and little-understood an area of the working of our remarkable and complex physiochemical systems. Providing that information has been a chief aim of this book.

It is equally my hope that a popular treatment of this sort will reach many of my fellow physicians who might not be aware of much of what has appeared about the subject in professional literature. There are so many papers published that it is unreasonable to expect every medical person to keep up with them all! This appendix is addressed primarily to those of my colleagues who find themselves convinced, or at least highly interested, by the material I have presented, and so wish to know more of specific techniques and approaches.

In this appendix, I shall deal with the details of nutrients for "supernutrition" and their food sources; methods of food testing; the clinical examination format, including environmental control and diagnostic and treatment procedures; proteolytic-enzyme therapy; and special techniques appropriate for hypo/hyperglycemia.

Nutrients for supernutrition

Supernutrition includes the use of the nutrients listed in Table A.1. Specific deficiencies first must be recognized and then treated accordingly. In the treatment of any deficiencies, one must remember

TABLE A.1. *Nutrients for Supernutrition and Their Food Sources*

Vitamins

Vitamin A	Thiamine (B_1)	Vitamin B_{12}	Inositol (In)
Vitamin D	Riboflavin (B_2)	Vitamin B_{15}	Para-aminobenzoic acid (PABA)
Vitamin E	Niacinamide (B_3)	Biotin (Bio)	Rutin (Ru)
Vitamin K	Pantothenic acid (B_5)	Folic acid (Fol)	Bioflavonoids
Ascorbic acid (C)	Vitamin B_6	Choline (Ch)	

Major Minerals

Calcium (Ca)	Potassium (K)	Sodium (Na)
Chlorine (Cl)	Magnesium (Mg)	Phosphate (PO_4)

Trace Minerals

Cobalt (Co)	Fluorine (F)	Manganese (Mn)	Zinc (Zn)
Chromium (Cr)	Iron (Fe)	Molybdenum (Mo)	
Copper (Cu)	Iodine (I)	Selenium (Se)	

Amino Acids

Isoleucine (Isol)	Methionine (Met)	Threonine (Thr)	Valine (Val)
Leucine (Leu)	Phenylalanine (Phe)	Tryptophan (Try)	Cystine (essential for some patients)
Lysine (Lys)			

Foods high in specific nutrients

Vitamin A

Beef liver	mackerel	spinach	carrots
melons	halibut	crab	beet greens
tomato	papaya	salmon	oysters
mustard greens	kale	grapefruit	cream cheese
swordfish	squash	sweet potato	

Vitamin C

beef liver	sweet potato	cabbage	strawberries
raspberries	oysters	alfalfa sprouts	spinach
avocado	blueberries	Brazil nuts	green pepper
collard	blackberries	banana	potato
tomato	citrus fruit	rose hips	pineapple
squash	mustard greens		

Vitamin D

beef liver	milk	tuna	chicken liver
sardines	salmon	egg yolk	herring

Vitamin E

cold-pressed oils	eggs	parsley	sweet potatoes	wheat germ

Vitamin F

vegetable oils	butter	sunflower seeds

Vitamin K

liver	soy	cauliflower
egg yolk	broccoli	green leafy vegetables

Thiamine

beef heart	cod	wheat	Brazil nuts	pineapple

B_1

beef liver	trout	rice	cashews
beef kidney	flounder	barley	pecans
milk	mackerel	peanuts	sesame seeds
crab	perch	soy	sunflower seeds
oysters	red snapper	pork liver	pumpkin

Riboflavin

beef	salmon	clams	Brazil nuts

B_2

beef kidney	trout	oysters	almonds
beef heart	cod	collard	beef liver
mackerel	mushrooms	chicken liver	perch

Pyridoxine

beef	halibut	crab	rice	peas

B_6

beef liver	mackerel	pork liver	prunes	soy
beef heart	salmon	pork heart	avocado	lentils
chicken	sardines	barley	Brazil nuts	peanuts
milk	tuna	wheat	lima beans	

B_{12}

beef	yogurt	sardines	egg
beef liver	milk	tuna	prunes
pork liver	cheddar cheese	cream cheese	

B_{15}

apricot kernels	rice bran	rice shoots	brewer's yeast	liver

Niacin

beef	cod	squash	dried apricot	peanuts
beef liver	perch	tomato	peach	almonds
beef kidney	trout	potato	avocado	papaya
pumpkin seeds	chicken	salmon	broccoli	watermelon
sunflower seeds	turkey	mackerel	collard	soy
sesame seeds	pork	sardines	mushrooms	wheat
pecans	clams	halibut	green beans	barley
cashews	oysters	haddock	lima beans	rice
brazil nuts	crab	strawberries	garbanzo beans	corn
boysenberries	shrimp	raspberries	peas	

Folic acid

beef liver	mackerel	barley	blackberries	almonds
beef heart	tuna	rice	avocado	pecans
turkey	peanuts	plums	walnuts	
cottage cheese	lima beans	raisins	dates	

TABLE A.1 (continued).

Pantothenic				
beef	salmon	clams	avocado	soy
acid	beef liver	mackerel	crab	pineapple
lentils	pork liver	sardines	mushrooms	bean sprouts
watermelon	chicken	lobster		
Inositol				
beef	chicken	rice	apple	
beef liver	salmon	peanuts	grapefruit	
pork	orange	strawberries	raisins	
Choline				
beef	egg	split peas	green beans	
garbanzo beans	beef liver	peanuts	bean sprouts	
pork liver	soy	milk	lentils	
Biotin				
beef	sardines	lima beans	garbanzo beans	avocado
beef liver	mackerel	split peas	lentils	grapefruit
pork liver	tuna	turnip greens	peanuts	watermelon
chicken	salmon	cauliflower	soy	almonds
eggs		mushrooms		
Rutin				
buckwheat	liver	eggs		
Para-aminobenzoic acid (PABA)				
beef liver	yogurt	wheat germ	green leafy vegetables	
beef heart	beef kidney			
Bioflavonoids				
lemon	lime	grapefruit	orange	red pepper
Zinc				
oysters	pumpkin seeds	grains	sunflower seeds	pork
Manganese				
egg yolk	grain	nuts	pineapple	sunflower seeds
Magnesium				
beef	salmon	barley	dried apricot	pecans
milk	flounder	rice	avocado	almonds
pork	tuna	peanuts	dates	cashews
chicken	crab	sesame	shrimp	brazil nuts
Potassium				
beef	cod	tomato	dates	sunflower seeds
beef liver	flounder	collard	papaya	Brazil nuts
milk	haddock	lima beans	avocado	pecans
turkey	salmon	split peas	apricots	almonds
pork	perch	peanuts	bananas	orange
sardines	clams	soy		

Calcium

beef liver	cheese	shrimp	turnip greens	sesame seeds
chicken liver	clams	mackerel	collard	Brazil nuts
milk	crab	sardines	mustard greens	almonds
yogurt	oysters	salmon		

Phosphorus

beef	milk	cod	crab	sesame seeds
beef liver	yogurt	flounder	soy	pecans
pork liver	cheese	haddock	rice	walnuts
chicken	salmon	perch	peanuts	cashews
turkey	mackerel	tuna	barley	almonds
eggs	sardines	shrimp	sunflower seeds	Brazil nuts
oysters	clams	lobster		

Iron

beef	clams	haddock	eggplant	Brazil nuts
beef liver	oysters	mackerel	tomato	sunflower seeds
beef kidney	shrimp	perch	garbanzo beans	walnuts
pork	sardines	tuna	lima beans	sesame seeds
pork liver	cod	salmon	soy	almonds
chicken	flounder	wheat	raisins	peanuts
dried apricot	prunes	pumpkin seeds		

Iodine

salmon	all oils	shredded wheat
turkey	butter	
rabbit	lard	

Copper

calf's liver	wheat germ	tea	Brazil nuts	sunflower seeds
lamb's liver	mushrooms	pork liver	filberts	walnuts
oysters	yeast			

Molybdenum

buckwheat	oats	wheat germ	barley	sunflower seeds
eggs	soybean	lima beans	lentils	liver

Selenium

brewer's yeast	garlic	liver	eggs	brown rice

Chronium

eggs	brewer's yeast	black pepper	liver	whole wheat bread
molasses	mushrooms	beef	beets	

that supernutrition involves a complete chain of some forty nutrients. These nutrients, such as vitamins, minerals, trace elements, amino acids, enzymes, and others, always work best as a team. Consequently, one nutrient added as a supplement to an individual's diet can bring no favorable effect unless the diet also contains adequate amounts of all the other nutrients, or unless they are available from the reserves of the person being treated. In short, the nutrient chain, which physicians use to treat degenerative and infectious diseases, is as strong as its weakest link. Every nutrient in the list acts like a gear in a complicated machine; there are no nutrients (gears) that are totally independent or dispensable in the human machine.

Methods of deliberate food testing

Foods can be accurately tested for twelve days, with a maximum of thirty days, after the four- or five-day period of avoidance. Each meal is a single food, raw, boiled, or baked, with nothing other than pure salt (preferably sea salt) added. Any water consumed or used in cooking should be nonchemically treated. Usually four test meals can be done a day by arranging an 8:30 P.M. meal, usually fruit. It is best that the first and second days of food testing be with foods not suspected as maladaptive reactors—those infrequently eaten by the patient. The third day of testing is the best time to do the stress test to determine biochemical abnormalities and deficiencies. On the fourth through seventh days, test less frequently used foods.

When testing one member of the food family, it is preferable to test all members of that family consecutively. On the morning of the eighth day of testing, start with the cereal-grain family and proceed consecutively with wheat, mature corn, fresh corn, oats, and rice. Wheat is tested as cooked whole-grain cereal, salted to taste, or as dry wheat-grain cereal. If wheat or other cereal grains give uncertain evidence on the first testing, test the same specific meal two or even three times to make sure. Mature corn is tested as cornmeal mush with corn syrup, salted to taste. Oats can be tested as oatmeal, salted to taste. Rye is not tested simply because it is so much like wheat. If wheat is positive, it is assumed that rye will also be positive and is not tested unless frequently used. Barley is a grain that is also very closely related to wheat and is not ordinarily tested unless there is a particular reason a specific person has been coming in contact with a great amount of barley. Certain alcoholic drinks and food substances contain large amounts of barley. If necessary, barley can be tested by cooking the grains into a cereal. Parenthetically, rice does not contain gluten; therefore, there is less of a reaction to rice than to wheat, barley, or corn. However, there are common molds in all the cereal grains, and for this reason any or all of them may cause a reaction.

Dairy products are then introduced, starting with pasteurized cow's milk. It is preferable that the milk come in glass bottles rather than plastic or wax cartons, since these substances may cause a reaction. However, this is not always practical; therefore, the milk should be tested in the container. Two glasses or more of milk are given for the test, then cheeses are tested. Usually American cheese and cheddar cheese are given in separate test meals. If there are other cheeses that are commonly used, they also are given a separate test meal. Each dairy product must be tested separately because the processing makes a difference whether or not reactions will occur. If cottage cheese is tested, it should be tested as dry cottage cheese without cream, unless it has already been demonstrated that there was no reaction to pasteurized cow's milk. If buttermilk is used, it should be given as a separate test. The same is true for butter.

Dairy products deserve some special attention. There are many people who were known to be reactive to milk as infants and children, but who in later years used milk and assumed they had outgrown their allergic reactions to all dairy products. This usually proves to be a mistake, and they are now highly reactive and addicted to a number of dairy products. Dairy products pose three problems:

1. allergic reaction;
2. galactosemic reactions in those in whom galactosemia has been demonstrated to be present (one out of five schizophrenics); and
3. lactase deficiency (70 percent in African Americans and 10 percent in Caucasians).

Those with gastrointestinal cereal-grain reactions run very high in lactase deficiency because of the damage that has occurred to the upper intestinal tract. The classic reaction occurring on a deliberate food test of dairy products due to lactase deficiency is gastrointestinal pain, diarrhea, and anxiety attacks occurring within one or two hours. The anxiety attack occurs because in the presence of low lactase, lactose ferments and produces lactic acid, which is absorbed into the blood and consequently ties up calcium magnesium. All dairy products (except cheddar cheese) contain lactose. The amount of galactose in butter is negligible. In cheeses and yogurt it is concentrated. Galactosemia is a condition in which liver, sometimes on an inherited basis, is unable to adequately change galactose (a relatively nonusable and, if present in high enough amounts, toxic sugar) into glucose. The first step in the metabolism of lactose is to split lactose into glucose and galactose. The second step changes the galactose into glucose. Therefore, galactosemic subjects should not consume milk or cheese (other than cheddar cheese). If the subject is not otherwise reactive to cheddar cheese, it is a suitable food for the galactosemic.

Meats, fish, vegetables, and fruits can usually be adequately determined on a one-test-meal basis. Fruits are best placed in the 8:00 P.M. to 8:30 P.M. meal. While testing the above-mentioned foods, it is important to keep in mind that it has been clinically discovered that there are many people who react to spray residues, as well as preservatives, additives, and food coloring. The only way to differentiate the noncontaminated food from the prepared or market food is to test the organic food; if no reaction occurs, test the market food or otherwise prepared food. From a practical standpoint it is not always possible to do this. However, it is the ideal and should be kept in mind. A person may be reacting to a food as tested from the usual market source, and yet not be reacting to foods grown under conditions under which preservatives, insecticide sprays, food colorings, or additives are not used. Another method is to test first the food as usually eaten; then, in those cases where reactions occur, test the organically grown foods. Moreover, in a case where there are reactions to a large number of foods, one begins to suspect a reaction to chemicals in the food instead of the food itself. In these cases, it is best to differentiate the food source.

Provocative testing of chemicals

Chemical extracts are prepared for sublingual or intradermal serial-dilution testing. Cat and dog dander, dust, molds, pollens, trees, and so forth can be tested by one of these methods. Food coloring can be tested in the home by placing the certified coloring in a glass of water and drinking the mixture. Red, yellow, and blue should be tested. Green need not be tested because it is a combination of yellow and blue. Pet allergies can be determined by holding the animal close to your nose and sniff-testing for three to five minutes. Dust allergies can be determined by vacuuming the house and seeing if a reaction develops during the process. A gas reaction is often suspected when symptoms develop during the preparation of a meal while cooking over a gas stove; this can be determined by lighting the burners and being near the stove for five or more minutes.

It must also be considered that fumes from the food being cooked are also a possible cause of symptoms, and these must be differentiated. Another way to test for petrochemical hydrocarbons is to stand behind a running automobile for three to five minutes to see if symptoms develop. Candles can be sniffed, as well as waxes, decorative kerosene lamps, and magic markers. There are numerous items in any home that are manufactured from petroleum products. All these are potential hazards for the petrochemical-hydrocarbon reactor. Plastics are made from hydrocarbons, and some very sensitive people are even known to react to foods stored in plastic containers or in plastic bags. All cosmetics and hair conditioners should be sniff tested. Clothes can be sniff tested after being bleached or washed, or the subject can be exposed to the laundry room during the bleaching process or washing process to determine a possible reaction to chorine and/or perfume. Placing volatile objects or substances in a glass jar, warming the contents with the jar closed, and then smelling the contents is a good way to sniff test.

As with foods, all chemicals should be tested after a four- to six-day period of abstinence from contact. The reason that there must be at least a four-day period of abstinence is that chemicals often carry the same quality of addiction as do foods. Reactions to petrochemical hydrocarbons can be just as serious as reactions to foods. In this respect, the most dangerous instrument in the home is the gas stove. Many people are chronically sick, either mentally or physically, due to exposure to the fumes from a gas stove or a gas- or oil-fired, hot-air heating system. Any gas pilot light from such units as a stove, hot-water heater, or home-heating unit that is within the living quarters or even on the same floor will contaminate the environment with petrochemical hydrocarbons. The problem of sensitivity to petrochemical hydrocarbons can reach into even more common aspects of one's environment; some patients have been known to react seriously to fumes from a newspaper or recently printed book. This type of reaction is due to hydrocarbons in the ink. Fumes of magic markers are particularly prone to give hydrocarbon reactions. Numerous children have become violently hyperactive after a single exposure to magic markers. Even preparations for chapped lips have petrochemical-hydrocarbon petroleum bases, as do many hair conditioners and perfumes. In light of the petrochemical-hydrocarbon pollution problem, it seems apparent that the patient's entire home should be surveyed for possible chemical contacts. In fact, after demonstrating a reaction to one petrochemical-hydrocarbon contact, a stove, for example, there is no real reason to continue to test for more maladaptive reactions. It is best right then and there to remove all possible petrochemical-hydrocarbon exposures, and keep them as minimal in amount and frequency as possible. Luckily, hydrocarbon reactors do not always react to plastics, which should, therefore, always be tested separately. You may find this difficult to believe, but natural pine and cedar relate to the petrochemical hydrocarbons and should also be tested separately as there may be a complete crossover between a gas stove and a pine panel door or a Christmas tree. Curiously, pine scented cleaners are particularly known for their production of serious reactions in susceptible persons.

The following may be helpful as a list of symptoms to look for during testing of foods and chemicals. A patient's food and chemical survey chart is also presented on pages 199–205.

Joints ache, pain, stiff, swelling, erythema, warmth, redness

Skin itching (local, general), scratching, moist, sweating, flushing, hives, pallor (white or ghostly)

Head pain headache (mild, moderate), severe migraine, ache, pressure, tight, exploding, throbbing, stabbing

Fatigue tired, generalized heaviness, sleepy, yawning, exhausted, fall asleep

Generalized dizzy, lightheaded, imbalance, staggering, vertigo, blackout, going to faint, chilly, cold, warmth, hot flashes

Depressed withdrawn, listless, vacant, dull faces, negative, indifferent, confused, dazed, depressed, crying, sobbing

Stimulated silly, intoxicated, grimacing, more alert, talkative, hyperactive, tense, restless, anxious, apprehensive, fear, panic, irritable, angry

Speech comprehension mentally sluggish, concentration poor, memory loss (acute), speech slurred, stammering, stuttering, speech paralysis, reads aloud poorly, reads without comprehension, hears without comprehension, math, spelling errors

Muscle muscle tremor, jerking, muscle cramps, spasms, pseudo-paralysis, weak

Contact poor contact, surroundings unreal, disoriented, catatonic, stuporous, false belief, delusion, hallucination; to wander in mind; false perception, suicidal, feel like hurting self, maniacal, very highly disturbed

Nasal sneezing, itching, rubbing, obstruction, discharge, postnasal drip, sinus discomfort, stuffy feeling

Throat, mouth itching, sore, tight, swollen, dysphagia, difficulty in swallowing, choking, weak voice, hoarse, salivation, mucus, metallic taste

Ears itching, full or blocked, erythema of pinna (reddening), tinnitis (ringing in ears), earache, hearing loss, hyperacusis (abnormal, sensitivity to sound)

Lungs, heart coughing, wheezing, reduced air flow, retracting, sob, heavy, tight, not enough air, hyperventilation (rapid breathing), chest pain, tachycardia (rapid pulse), palpitations (rapid, violent, or throbbing pulses), premature ventricular contractions (PVCs)

Eyes itch, burn, pain, lacrimation (tearing), allergic shiners, feel heavy, red

Vision blurring, acuity decreased, spots, flashes, darker, vision loss, photophobia (brighter), diplopia (double vision), dyslexia (difficulty reading—transposition of similar letters; letters or words becoming small or large; words moving around)

G-U voided, mild urge, frequency, urgency, pressure, painful or difficult urination, dysuria (genital itch)

G-I (Abdomen) nausea, belching, full, bloated, vomiting, pressure, pain, cramps, flatus, rumbling, bowel movement (BM), diarrhea, gall bladder, symptoms, hunger, thirst, hyperacidity

Muscles tight, stiff, ache, sore, pain, neck, trapezius, upper-lower back, upper-lower extremities

FOOD AND CHEMICAL SURVEY TO DETERMINE CONTACTS WITH BASIC FOODS AND CHEMICALS

For the patient to fill out

CIRCLE ALL ITEMS USED, CHECK USE AND REACTIONS, AND GIVE COMMENTS	DAILY	3 x a week	1–2 x a week	SELDOM		Binges	Love	Crave	Feel better	Picked up	More energetic	More alert, etc.	Makes me ill	Dislike		
	USE					REACTIONS									COMMENTS	TEST INFORMATION
Wheat																
bread, crackers																
cake, cookies																
spaghetti, macaroni																
pizza, pasta																
cereal (hot/cold)																
buckwheat																
Rye																
crackers																
cereal																
bread																
Oats (oatmeal)																
hot/cold cereals																
cookies																
Barley																
malt																
malted milk																
Corn																
corn sugar																
syrup																
oil (margarine)																
fresh corn																
Rice																
Legumes																
pea, green																
lima beans																
gr. beans (string)																
peanuts																
soy (beans, sauce)																
lentils																
navy beans																
Milk																
powdered skim																

CIRCLE ALL ITEMS USED, CHECK USE AND REACTIONS, AND GIVE COMMENTS	USE					REACTIONS									COMMENTS	TEST INFORMATION
	DAILY	3 x a week	1–2 x a week	SELDOM		Binges	Love	Crave	Feel better	Picked up	More energetic	More alert, etc.	Makes me ill	Dislike		
Milk *(continued)*																
ice cream																
yogurt																
Cheese																
cottage																
cream																
American																
swiss																
cheddar																
others																
Beef (veal)																
steak																
roast																
hamburger																
Fish																
salmon																
catfish																
perch																
swordfish																
Eggs																
Vegetables																
beet																
spinach																
mustard greens																
turnip																
radish																
cabbage																
cauliflower																
broccoli																
brussels sprouts																
tomato																
potato																
sweet potato																

CIRCLE ALL ITEMS USED, CHECK USE AND REACTIONS, AND GIVE COMMENTS	DAILY	3 x a week	1–2 x a week	SELDOM	Binges	Love	Crave	Feel better	Picked up	More energetic	More alert, etc.	Makes me ill	Dislike		
	USE				REACTIONS									COMMENTS	TEST INFORMATION
red pepper (hot)															
carrot															
celery															
parsnips															
green pepper															
lettuce															
asparagus															
Fruit															
apple															
pear															
orange															
lemon															
grapefruit															
apricot															
cherry															
peach															
plum															
date															
banana															
grape															
pineapple															
blueberry															
cranberry															
strawberry															
blackberry															
raspberry															
canned fruit in syrup															
Gourds															
cantaloupe															
honeydew															
watermelon															
cucumber															
squash															
pumpkin															

CIRCLE ALL ITEMS USED, CHECK USE AND REACTIONS, AND GIVE COMMENTS	DAILY	3 x a week	1–2 x a week	SELDOM		Binges	Love	Crave	Feel better	Picked up	More energetic	More alert, etc.	Makes me ill	Dislike		
	USE					REACTIONS									COMMENTS	TEST INFORMATION
Nuts & Seeds																
cashew nut																
pistachio nut																
sunflower seeds																
pumpkin seeds																
almond																
walnut																
pecan																
coconut																
Miscellaneous																
olives																
mushroom																
chocolate																
coffee																
tea																
baker's yeast																
brewer's yeast																
honey (clover)																
Other																

Being late for a meal or missing a meal completely makes me ill. ( ) Yes ( ) No

Eating relieves the symptoms from late or missed meals. ( ) Yes ( ) No

The food(s) that give the greatest or quickest relief of these fasting symptoms is/are:

CHEMICAL ODORS, VAPORS, FUMES

In your home is there a gas or electric stove? Kitchen range?

Refrigerator? Water heater?

Heating system (gas, electric, oil, etc.)?

For the patient to fill out

CIRCLE ALL ITEMS USED, CHECK USE AND REACTIONS, AND GIVE COMMENTS	DAILY	3 x a week	1–2 x a week	SELDOM	Binges	Love	Crave	Feel better	Picked up	More energetic	More alert, etc.	Makes me ill	Dislike		
	USE				REACTIONS									COMMENTS	TEST INFORMATION
leaking natural gas															
auto exhaust															
bus exhaust															
truck exhaust															
floor wax															
furniture wax															
polish (all types)															
oven cleaner															
window cleaner															
brush cleaner															
moth balls															
magic marker															
freshly printed:															
newspapers															
magazines															
cigar smoke															
cigarette smoke															
pipe smoke															
gasoline															
black top roads (tar)															
paint thinner															
paint remover															
freshly painted room															
rubber tires															
rubber gloves															
plastic-shower curtain															
disinfectant															
air freshener															
detergent															
ammonia															
chlorine															
cleaning agent															
deodorant spray															

CIRCLE ALL ITEMS USED, CHECK USE AND REACTIONS, AND GIVE COMMENTS	DAILY	3 x a week	1–2 x a week	SELDOM		Binges	Love	Crave	Feel better	Picked up	More energetic	More alert, etc.	Makes me ill	Dislike		
	USE					REACTIONS									COMMENTS	TEST INFORMATION
hair spray																
perfume																
glue - cement																
medications																

DOCTOR'S CHECKLIST

Patient to check items he or she is aware of

CIRCLE ALL ITEMS USED, CHECK USE AND REACTIONS, AND GIVE COMMENTS	DAILY	3 x a week	1–2 x a week	SELDOM		Binges	Love	Crave	Feel better	Picked up	More energetic	More alert, etc.	Makes me ill	Dislike		
	USE					REACTIONS									COMMENTS	TEST INFORMATION
Chemicals																
auto exhaust																
ethanol																
maltox																
isotox																
plastic																
chlorine																
Molds																
alternaria																
aspergillis																
homodendrium																
Animals																
cat																
dog																
horse																
other																
Certified Food Color																
red																
blue																
yellow																

CIRCLE ALL ITEMS USED, CHECK USE AND REACTIONS, AND GIVE COMMENTS	DAILY	3 x a week	1–2 x a week	SELDOM		Binges	Love	Crave	Feel better	Picked up	More energetic	More alert, etc.	Makes me ill	Dislike		
	USE					REACTIONS									COMMENTS	TEST INFORMATION
Miscellaneous																
tobacco																
dust																
cane sugar																
magic marker																
chap stick																

ALCOHOLIC BEVERAGES

Information on this subject is important even though you may take only an occasional social drink.

Did alcohol at any time in your life cause symptoms that it no longer produces? ( ) Yes ( ) No

	Immediate Symptoms		**Delayed Symptoms**		**Describe**	**Test Information**
	Yes	**No**	**Yes**	**No**		
beer						
cocktails						
gin						
rum						
scotch						
vodka						
wine						
rye						
bourbon						
others						

Medical and technical information on a clinical examination format

Environmental control

There are several environmental control units in hospitals in which the patient should be isolated from his commonly contacted chemicals and supervised in the food-avoidance period and testing. It would be ideal for state hospitals and private psychiatric hospitals to have such environmental control units. At present, none are available specifically for psychiatric patients.

If the patient is at home, individual reactions to, for example, petrochemical hydrocarbons from gas stoves, synthetic rugs, synthetic clothing, cats, dogs, and so on are examined. The home is then sufficiently cleared of these items to make it environmentally appropriate for the avoidance period of the test. Frequently, all gas pilot lights have to be turned off. Sometimes an air filter has to be provided for the bedroom. The pillow on which the patient sleeps needs to be considered to make sure no reaction is occurring to foam rubber, Dacron®, or feathers. When the patient is away from home, a suitable motel, hotel, or efficiency apartment is arranged. Chemical cleaning agents or toilet-bowl chemicals should not be used for the period the patient is in these quarters. Sometimes an air filter is necessary for the room.

Diagnostic and treatment procedures

Avoidance period

Fasting is required, giving only spring, well, or distilled water to which the patient has been tested and found not to be reactive. It is important not to have fluorine or chlorine in the water since some react to these chemicals. The patient comes to the office eight hours a day on Wednesday, Thursday, and Friday of this fast and is at home or in the motel on Saturday and Sunday. These two days the patient is on his own, although the doctor is always on call. Symptoms have usually subsided substantially or even ceased by the fourth day of the fast. In some cases, vitamins and minerals are given intravenously for the first, second, and third days of the fast and only occasionally extended to the fourth or fifth day. The IV shots consist of 12½ grams of vitamin C, 1,000 milligrams of B_6, 1,250 milligrams of B_5, 2 grams of magnesium sulfate or chloride and 10 cc of calphasan or calcium gluconate. Sometimes 5 cc of B-complex vitamins is also given intramuscularly. The IV is given over a thirty-minute period or more near the end of the day. In few very disturbed patients, the IV is given two times per day for three days. Sometimes 5,000 units of heparin are placed in the IV. On the evening of the first or sometimes the second day of the fast, the patient clears his colon by taking two tablespoons of Milk of Magnesia or an ascorbate (vitamin C) flush. The ascorbate flush is the most effective and consists of two teaspoons of sodium ascorbate (vitamin C) in half a glass of water every fifteen minutes for four hours. This produces an intestinal flush as well as maximum absorption of vitamin C. Some have symptoms markedly reduced during the ascorbate flush. If desired, fructose can be added to the sodium ascorbate to increase tolerance. Even if the patient vomits during this ascorbate flush, he is asked to continue the process for four hours. Some patients sip the sodium ascorbate over a fifteen-minute period rather than drink it all at once, in order to avoid vomiting.

Sodium ascorbate is more suitable to the withdrawal phase of addictions simply because it is alkaline; that is, it helps reduce the acidosis inherent in the withdrawal phase. An added relief value can occur if the following is added to each dose of vitamin C during the withdrawal phase: 500 milligrams of B_6, 100 to 500 milligrams of B_2, and ten to fifteen 750-milligram capsules of amino acid. The best amino acids for this purpose are not from food sources but come from bacteria. Other symptom-relieving agents or methods available include:

1. One teaspoon of sodium bicarbonate can be taken whenever needed. This is best provided as sodium and potassium bicarbonate in a ratio of 2:1.
2. One-tenth to ¼ cc of heparin can be taken sublingually whenever needed up to six times a day (can be used subcutaneously, if desired, for quick and more effective relief). Heparin comes in 5,000 units per cc and 10,000 units per cc and can be obtained from either beef or pork sources. These are all suitable. Substantially higher doses of heparin are necessary when it is used as an anticoagulant instead of simply an anti-inflammatory agent as in this case.
3. One-fourth to ½ cc of procaine (2 percent) taken orally, subcutaneously, or intramuscularly can also help relieve symptoms. This can be used as often as desired for its anti-inflammatory value. Procaine should not be considered a drug, but is a precursor to para-aminobenzoic acid and DEAE, which is a natural occurring antidepressant. For some combination of reasons, procaine has virtually an equal value to proteolytic enzymes, such as heparin, in its anti-inflammatory value. It has been used for years in Romania and other European countries to retard the aging process and undoubtedly works because of its anti-inflammatory value in reducing reactions to foods and chemicals.
4. Breathing pure oxygen (O_2) for ten minutes or more will often reduce symptoms.
5. Breathing 5 percent carbon dioxide (CO_2) and 95 percent oxygen is about twice as effective as oxygen alone.
6. Breathing 30 percent nitrous oxide plus 5 percent carbon dioxide plus 65 percent oxygen for several minutes is quite effective in relieving symptoms.

Not every person voluntarily agrees to fast, and some are not physically suited to it. For example, markedly malnourished patients, severe asthmatics, epileptics, and some others may be judged as not suitable for a fast. Those not being fasted have some alternatives:

1. For the five-day avoidance period, test foods that are infrequently used and do not relate to food families commonly used by the patient. This testing will not be as reliable as the testing after the avoidance period because it is clouded by the emerging withdrawal symptoms. Any food tests that are questioned can be given again at a later date.
2. Eat freely of foods not commonly used, such as rutabaga, turnip greens, and olives, or eat watermelon only. If on the initial test meal the patient does not react to watermelon with symptoms of hyperglycemia or other symptoms, it is a good single food for the avoidance period, since it contains potassium, which tends to be depleted during this time. Carrot juice is also good for this purpose.

No matter what system is being used, whether fasting or eating foods that are not commonly used, the blood sugar is taken each morning for days one, two, and three. Sometimes hypoglycemia is sufficiently severe that it is best to abandon the fast and start feeding the patient uncommonly used foods.

There are special considerations that should be observed during the avoidance period. Diabetics should be tested under medical supervision. Clinical diabetics not on insulin can be fasted by monitoring saliva pH, urine for pH and ketones, and blood sugar on a four-hour-basis day and night. Whenever saliva is below 6.4 or the urine shows ketones or a pH below 6, one teaspoon of alkali salts is given in a glass of water. The alkali salts are sodium and potassium bicarbonate in a ratio of 2:1. Saliva pH is monitored with Hydron paper. A double-cartridge disposer is used with a pH of 5.2 to 6.6 and the other side a pH of 6 to 8. Normal saliva pH is 6.4 to 6.8 in a nonreactive, nonaddictive state. During addictive withdrawal and also at the time of acute allergic and allergic-like reactions, the saliva pH characteristically drops below 6.4. Monitoring of the urine can be done by the Ames N-Multistick, which will give the pH, protein, glucose, ketones, bilirubin, blood, nitrite, and urobilinogen in the urine. The Ames Keto-Diastix is also suitable for providing a reading on the ketones and glucose. The Keto-Stix provides a reading only on the ketones.

Insulin-dependent diabetics, whether maturity-onset or juvenile-onset, need special medical attention. Some maturity-onset diabetics who have not been ketoacidosis-prone can be fasted under medical monitoring. Insulin-dependent, juvenile diabetics cannot be fasted. In those cases that cannot be fasted, the initial reliance of reactivity to a food or substance comes from the intradermal, serial dilution provocative test supplemented by information from the cytotoxic test, RAST test, and sniff test. Insulin-dependent diabetics must have an Eyetone or Stak-Tek instrument for use at home and monitor all meals before and one hour after tests. Monitoring of blood sugar in the morning before feeding and before giving insulin soon reveals whether a true insulin dependence is available or not. Two-thirds of insulin-dependent, maturity-onset diabetics are found not to be insulin-dependent, and some diagnoses as insulin-dependent, juvenile diabetics are found to instead be maturity-onset and not insulin-dependent. When insulin is used, it is given in two or preferably three dosages of regular insulin or combined with NPH insulin.

Epileptics should be left on their medication and usually are not fasted, since a drop in blood sugar and the cerebral irritation of withdrawal may evoke seizures. Epileptics are as carefully monitored as diabetics.

Asthmatics with a history of acute attacks are best not fasted and must be carefully monitored. They should have bronchial dilators available at all times.

Testing period

Three meals a day, five days a week, are tested in the clinic. One meal is tested in the evening at home and four meals a day at home on weekends. Those tests at the office are the frequently used foods to which a reaction may be anticipated; those tested at home are the least frequently used foods with the least chance of a reaction. On the home tests, the patient monitors and records his symptoms and pulse changes. He then turns this report into the physician. If the test is a serious reactor, it is retested in the office with the blood sugar monitored. In the office testing, the blood sugar is taken one hour after each test meal. If symptoms are severe before this hour, the blood sugar is taken after a half hour, and if they are severe after this hour, it is taken again at one and a half hours. If the blood sugar is beyond 160 milligrams percent on any test, the blood sugar is taken again before the next meal. No test meals are given unless or until the blood sugar is 120 milligrams percent or below. An objective observer records symptoms during the test, and the patient records the symptoms and pulse changes. A normal baseline pulse may range from 60 (an athletic person) to 85 (a nonathletic person). Marked shifts up or down from a pretest base line are significant. The pulse is tested for a full minute.

If and when symptoms occur during food testing, inhalation testing, sublingual testing, or intradermal provocative testing that are sufficiently severe to demand relief, there are several possibilities including:

1. pure O_2 for several minutes;
2. 95 percent O_2 plus 5 percent CO_2 for several minutes;
3. 30 percent N_2O plus 65 percent O_2 plus 5 percent CO_2 for several minutes;
4. 1 teaspoon of alkali salts in a glass of water (sodium and potassium bicarbonate in a 2:1 ratio);
5. ¼ to ½ cc heparin (sublingual or subcutaneous);
6. ¼ to ½ cc 2 percent procaine hydrochloride (sublingual or intramuscular);
7. exercise to oxygenate tissues; and
8. in case of acute psychotic or migraine reactions, 44.6 mEq sodium bicarbonate IV and intravenous vitamins, minerals,

> and heparin consisting of 12½ grams to 25 grams sodium ascorbate, 1,000 milligrams of B_6, 1,250 milligrams of B_5, 5,000 units of heparin, 2 grams of magnesium chloride, and 10 cc of calphasan diluted in the 100 to 200 cc normal saline can be useful.

When acute reactions occur, the urine is collected three hours after the test meal and monitored for vitamin C by using the Ames C-Stix. Any level below 40 milligrams percent is abnormally low. I have found some foods that are severely reacted to in patients that give a reading of 0 to 5 milligrams percent. Moreover, a large percentage of patients have 0 milligrams percent of vitamin C spillage when allergically reacting to several foods. Vitamin C deficiency is established as a result of allergic reactions to these specific foods. A patient reacting to these foods is rocking in and out of vitamin C deficiency.

Stress day

The stress day is usually the third or fifteenth day of the program. The purpose of this is to place the patient under the stress of reactions to foods in order to discover any further disordered body chemistry. All day the patient eats only symptom-reactive foods, smokes cigarettes if he wants, and takes 10 grams of tryptophan in three divided doses during the day. The tryptophan is an amino acid that makes a special demand for B_6 and will bring out the evidence of B_6 deficiency when even a borderline deficiency occurs. This test is patterned after the tryptophan loading test which is a standard accepted test for the discovery of B_6 deficiency. A twenty-four-hour urine is collected and tested for:

- spillage of kynurenic acid and xanthurenic acid to detect B_6 deficiency (B_6 deficiency or disordered utilization occurs in approximately 75 percent of the patients);
- spillage of formiminoglutamic acid (FIGLU test) to determine folic-acid deficiency;

- spillage of vitamin C; and
- spillage of amino acids to determine amino-acid deficiency.

The morning after the stress day, a blood sample is drawn and tested for complete blood count, alkaline phosphatase, bilirubin (total), BUN, cholesterol, triglycerides, creatinine, LDH, SGOT, SGPT, uric acid, CPK, free fatty acids, sometimes histamines, B_{12}, iron, magnesium, thiamine (transketolase), thyroid group (T3, T4, and free thyroxine), and an immunoprotein panel (including IgM, IgA, IgG, C-3 complement, Alpha-2 macroglobulin, albumin, transferring, Alpha-1-antitrypsin, Alpha-1-acid glycoprotein, C-4 complement, ceruloplasmin, and haptoglobin).

There are several other tests, unrelated to the stress day, which are done:

1. RAST, for single antigens to several foods, grasses, dog and cat dander, pollen, and house dust.
2. PRIST, for IgE.
3. Cytotoxic test for microscopic evidence of the blood reacting to foods, chemicals, and inhalants.
4. Sublingual, serial-dilution provocative testing used for a few items that for special cases cannot be tested in other ways.
5. Sniff provocative testing for a few chemical items such as petrochemical hydrocarbons.
6. Intradermal, serial-dilution provocative testing used as a major type testing in patients who for some reason cannot be tested with deliberate provocative food testing. These include insulin-dependent diabetics and some epileptics. This method of testing is also used to determine the optimum immunological dosage for infectious agents, molds, fungi, and similar items.
7. Chemical urinalysis using the Ames N-Multistix. This is used repeatedly during the withdrawal phase and test phases to determine changes occurring during these stress

periods. It includes pH, protein, glucose, ketones, bilirubin, blood, nitrite, and urobilinogen.

8. Hair test biopsy. This is to test for calcium, magnesium, sodium, potassium, copper, zinc, phosphorus, iron, manganese, chromium, lithium, selenium, nickel, tin, aluminum, cobalt, molybdenum, and the toxic metals lead, mercury, arsenic, and cadmium.
9. Bacterial cultures, identification and antibiotic sensitivity from such areas as the throat, nose, sinuses, prostate, vagina, and skin when judged as needed. This is in preparation for antibiotic treatment. Sometimes autogenous vaccines are prepared. Stock bacterial vaccines are routinely used after intradermal serial-dilution provocative testing to determine optimum dosage for the vaccine.
10. Culture and identification of fungi, especially *Candida albicans*, from such areas as the nose, throat, armpits, vagina, rectum, and any lesions of the skin or nails. If *Candida albicans* or other fungi are present, the patient is treated with nystatin or other appropriate antifungal medication. *Candida albicans* is often found in the throat or rectum, giving evidence of a gastrointestinal infection. This is treated vigorously over a period of a month with oral tablets and an oral solution rinse of the mouth and throat. *Candida albicans* is considered a hidden culprit, which can set the stage for numerous reactions; it should always be tested for and never missed by an orthomolecular psychiatrist.
11. Dark-field microscopic study of the blood for *Progenitor cryptocides* reveals the degree of infection with this microorganism. BCG vaccine is given as a stock vaccine against this organism. In some patients it is important to add to this an autogenous vaccine prepared from a culture made from the urine or feces. James Papyes cultured this pleomorphic organism from the brains of schizophrenics and observed its characteristic of parasitizing red blood cells. It is believed that episodic flare-ups of cerebral in-

fection with this microbe superimposed on reactions to foods and chemicals is central in the deteriorating process of schizophrenia. This microbe is known to be carcinogenic and is routinely found in cancerous tumors.

12. The Heidelberg gastrograph used to produce evidence of the pH of the stomach and of the small intestine. A small number of people have little or no acid in their stomachs. This determination demonstrates digestive malfunction for proteins and indicates the need for acid supplementation with meals. A low alkaline state in the small intestine after a test meal of symptom-producing food indicates poor pancreatic function and suggests the need for alkali and pancreatic enzymes after meals.
13. A parallel glucose and insulin determination is made in certain cases to determine if insulin is adequate in response to meals. This can be an aid in determining true insulin dependence.

In treating those who desire a vegetarian diet, special considerations are necessary. Vegetarians are just as prone to food allergies as nonvegetarians. They, too, become addicted (allergic) to their most frequently eaten foods. As with the beef and pork eater who becomes allergic to beef and pork, so, too, the milk, wheat, soybean, and egg eater can become addicted to these foods. Classical vegetarians are heavy users of cereal grains and often rely on wheat gluten as a basic source of protein; this leaves the vegetarian who may be genetically programmed as a reactor to wheat in a vulnerable position, since she is more prone to use wheat and other gluten-bearing cereal grains. In my studies, wheat is seen to be the highest maladaptive reacting substance, especially in evoking mental symptoms. In vulnerable persons, I have clinically evoked full-blown psychosis with a test of gluten steaks. Likewise, I have evoked serious physical and mental symptoms on test exposures to soy or milk in those addicted to these items. The use of organic foods is not a guarantee against addiction even though such foods contain fewer chemicals to react to and provide, by and large, a superior supply of necessary nutrients.

The vegetarian should be tested widely for specific foods within commonly eaten family groups. By testing broadly within these family groups, vegetarians can often find suitable nonreactive foods. It is well to include in the diet rare types of greens and even an assortment of wild greens. It is also advisable to include comfrey as a cooked green or in a green drink. Greens are a valuable source of many minerals, vitamins, and proteins and thus should always be part of a rotation diet.

For the vegetarian who is broadly reactive to his commonly eaten foods, there may need to be a temporary daily use of specifically nutritious foods to which there is no reaction while rotating all other foods. If tolerated, ten or more alfalfa tablets should be used three times a day on the legume day. Also, if tolerated, brewer's yeast or a similar dry yeast should be used in dosages of 1 or 2 tablespoons three times a day on a suitable day of rotation. For the strict vegetarian who wishes to avoid beef or pork products as amino acid supplements or enzyme supplements, there are amino acids available from soy, whey, alfalfa, and bacterial sources. There are enzymes available from the mold *Aspergillus*, bromelain from pineapple, and papain from papaya.

Examples of Commonly Recommended Nutrients for Severely Allergic Patients

Nutrient	*Adult*	*Child (50 to 80 lbs.)*
Ascorbic acid powder	1 tsp. powder, t.i.d.	½ tsp., t.i.d.
or		
Sodium ascorbate as powder 4 g/tsp.	Bowel tolerance	Bowel tolerance
Pyridozine or	500 mg, t.i.d.	100 mg, t.i.d.
Pyridoxal-5-phosphate	50 mg, t.i.d.	25 mg, t.i.d.
Riboflavin	500 mg, t.i.d.	100 mg, t.i.d.
Pantothenic acid	500 mg, t.i.d.	100 mg, t.i.d.
Thiamine	500 mg, t.i.d.	100 mg, t.i.d.

Niacinamide or niacin	500 mg, t.i.d.	100 mg, t.i.d.
Para-aminobenzoic acid	500 mg, t.i.d.	100 mg, t.i.d.
Folic acid	400 mcg, t.i.d.	400 mcg, t.i.d.
Vitamin E	400 units, t.i.d.	400 units once/day
Vitamin A	10,000 units, t.i.d.	10,000 units once/day
Vitamin D	400 units, t.i.d.	400 units once/day
L-Glutamine	500 mg, t.i.d.	500 mg once to twice/day
L-Tryptophan	1,500 mg at bedtime; repeat in one hour if needed for sleep	500 to 1,500 mg at bedtime

Note: Dosages may vary greatly among different individuals.

L-Glutamine is used routinely. L-Tryptophan is used only for insomnia. Be sure the pyridoxine and riboflavin supplements are being taken when tryptophan is being used since it can cause B_6 deficiency.

An acidophilus capsule or tablet may be taken once a day as a minimum with each meal, if indicated. A freeze-dried, nonmilk source is available for milk reactors.

A good source of vitamins A and D is Hain's cod liver oil concentrate, which provides 16,600 units vitamin A and 1,660 units vitamin D per teaspoon. Start with 2 teaspoons, BID, for six weeks, followed by 1 teaspoon, BID, thereafter. Children are treated according to the percentage of their body weight compared to an adult's.

The B-complex vitamins can best be obtained in capsules of 500 and 100 milligrams. If there is an allergic reaction to the gelatin capsule (pork or beef source) the contents can be removed from the capsule. Seldom do people react to gelatin capsules even if they react to beef or pork. If the capsules contain bicarbonate as a filler, take them thirty to forty-five minutes after the meal; this is important because bicarbonate interferes with the gastric phase of digestion but aids the intestinal phase of digestion. Tablets without corn, sugar, or color are available but contain a filler called avacid (made from cotton or wood) to which some people react. Vitamin E should be synthetic, or else rotate wheat and soy sources if not reactive to these.

Examples of Commonly Recommended Nutrients

Nutrient	*Adult*	*Child (50 to 80 lbs.)*
Magnesium	75 mg, t.i.d.	75 mg once or twice/day
Zinc	10 mg, t.i.d.	10 mg once or twice/day
Manganese	10 mg, t.i.d.	10 mg once or twice/day
Chromium	1 mg, t.i.d.	1 mg once or twice/day
Potassium	150 mg, t.i.d.	150 mg once or twice/day
Copper	5 mg, t.i.d.	5 mg once or twice/day
Selenium	100 mg, t.i.d.	100 mg once or twice/day

When the hair-test biopsy is normal or in excess, no mineral is given. Magnesium and zinc are given even if in normal limits. When the hair reveals deficiency, then minerals are given in the amounts indicated. Repeat hair test twice a year to monitor minerals. Serum studies of zinc, chromium, magnesium, and calcium are also done. Any deficiency in serum or hair is honored with preference being given to serum. Calcium may be deficient in the serum when high in the hair.

Prescription, mineralized drinking water is a good way to give the minerals. They are placed in drinking water, and ten glasses for an adult and five glasses for a child provide the desired amount of minerals. The minerals are placed in five gallons of water. As many as possible are in the form of bicarbonate, and the amount of C that will turn these bicarbonates into ascorbates is added to the water. Those not available as bicarbonate are used as salts of the minerals. Minerals are also available as chelates of soy amino acids. Some, however, cannot tolerate the soy.

Proteolytic enzyme therapy

Proteolytic enzymes digest proteins into amino acids. Without adequate proteolytic enzymes, amino-acid deficiency results. The guiding principle of treatment is to be sure to use an adequate amount for maximum inhibition of inflammation. The schedule can vary from three to six doses in twenty-four hours, and is usually best to have at least one dose during the night, although some will do well with three daytime doses.

1. *At the beginning of the meal:* If the gastric acid has been demonstrated to be low, then give glutamic acid HCL and/or betaine HCL, or a digestive enzyme tablet containing these plus pepsin and pancreatic concentrate.
2. *End of meal:* One or two tablets, 225 to 400 milligrams, pancreas compound.
3. *Thirty to forty-five minutes after the meal:* One tablet pancreas compound (sometimes two tablets may be indicated): one tablet bromelain with papain; 10 to 20 grams of sodium bicarbonate or ¼ to ½ teaspoon of sodium bicarbonate and potassium bicarbonate (⅔; ⅓).
4. *At bedtime:* Two tablets of pancreas compound; two bromelain tablets with papain.

Maintain this program for two to four months and then reduce it according to the patient's needs. The sodium bicarbonate is necessary to produce the alkali required for activation of the pancreatic enzymes. It is given thirty minutes after the meal so as not to interfere with the acid gastric phase of digestion. The alkali should be given earlier than a half hour if epigastric discomfort accompanies eating. Bear in mind that the goal is to have the local intestinal alkalinity high enough to provide an alkaline medium for the function of the proteolytic digestive process, as well as providing absorption of proteolytic enzymes and systemic postmeal activation of the systemic proteolytic enzyme pool so as to prevent kinin-mediated inflammatory reactions from occurring in response to the absorbed foods.

Case histories

I. Catatonia Schizophrenia—Woman: Age 26

A. Test meal of cheddar cheese

Test for cheddar cheese before proteolytic enzymes
Initial Reaction: Markedly sweating hands followed by tension which progressed to rigid catatonia.

Test for cheddar cheese after proteolytic enzymes

1. 1,670 milligrams concentrated pancreatic enzymes in enteric-coated tablets. Glutamic acid HCL and pepsin also in the nonenteric-coated part of the tablet. Blood sugar 75 milligrams percent.
2. Thirty minutes after step one, blood sugar was 80 milligrams percent.
3. Fifty minutes after step one, 1,670 milligrams concentrated pancreatic enzymes in enteric-coated tablets were given.
4. Fifty-five minutes after step one, she ate one pound of cheddar cheese.
5. Thirty minutes after the test meal, ¼ teaspoon sodium bicarbonate plus potassium bicarbonate (⅔, ⅓) was given. Blood sugar was still stable at 80 milligrams percent.
6. One hour after test meal, blood sugar was 80 milligrams percent.

Results of test: No tension or catatonia. She was mentally clear and alert. The only symptom was minor sweating of hands.

It is important to note that in the treatment of a severe degenerative mental disease like schizophrenia, the particular dosage of pancreatic enzymes is often increased. The following case histories give the exact clinical dosages as well as the treatment procedures.

B. Test meal of dairy butter and Irish potatoes

Test for dairy butter before proteolytic enzymes
Initial reaction: Initial nausea and vomiting. Blood sugar 110 milligrams percent

Test for Irish potato before proteolytic enzymes
Initial reaction: Hands cold, tense and nervous. Feels hot; breathing labored.

Test for dairy butter and Irish potato after proteolytic enzymes

1. Blood sugar was 80 milligrams percent. Symptom-free. Administered 1,670 milligrams of pancreatic enzymes in enteric-coated tablets plus glutamic acid HCL, betaine HCL, and pepsin.
2. Thirty minutes after step one, blood sugar was 80 milligrams percent and she was symptom-free. Test meal of Irish potato and dairy butter given.
3. Thirty minutes after the test meal, ¼ teaspoon of alkali salts were given. Blood sugar was 90 milligrams percent.
4. One hour after the test meal, blood sugar was 100 milligrams percent.

Results of test: The only symptom was very slight nausea.

C. Test meal of peanuts

Test for peanuts before and after proteolytic enzymes
Initial reaction: Irritability, depression, crying, and dissociation. A test meal after proteolytic enzymes was on the order of 1,670 milligrams of pancreatic enzyme concentrate forty minutes before the meal, and another 1,670 milligrams at the time of the test meal. The blood sugar remained stable.

Results of test: The only symptom was slight sweating of the hands.

D. Test meal of beef

Test for beef before and after proteolytic enzymes
Initial reaction: Tension, a desire not to talk, a wish to be alone, feeling like screaming. The test meal using proteolytic enzymes was on the order of 1,670 milligrams pancreatic enzyme concentrate plus glutamic acid HCL, betaine HCL, and pepsin before the meal followed by ¼ teaspoon alkali salts thirty minutes after the meal.

Results of test: No symptoms developed.

II. Chronic Schizoaffective Reaction—Woman: Age 27

A. Test meal of raisins

Test for raisins before proteolytic enzymes
Initial reaction: One hour after test meal for raisins, the blood sugar was 400 milligrams percent (severe diabetic reaction). Symptoms were marked tension, trembling, irritability, and unprovoked anger at mother.

Test for raisins after proteolytic enzymes

1. Symptom-free. Blood sugar 100 milligrams percent. A test meal was on the order of 1,670 milligrams pancreatic enzyme concentrate in enteric-coated tablets plus the glutamic acid HCL, betain HCL, and pepsin.
2. Thirty minutes after step one, blood sugar was 100 milligrams percent. Symptom-free. A test meal on the order of 1,670 milligrams of pancreatic enzyme concentrate and other items was given as in step one. Meal of raisins given.
3. Thirty minutes after test meal, blood sugar was 160 milligrams percent. Symptom-free. A quarter of a teaspoon of sodium bicarbonate was given.
4. One hour after test meal, blood sugar was 120 milligrams percent. Symptom-free.

Results of test: No symptoms developed. Blood sugar remained normal.

B. Test meal of pineapple

Test for pineapple before proteolytic enzymes
Initial reaction: Blood sugar was 260 milligrams percent (normal range: up to 160 milligrams percent). No subjective or objective symptoms observed.

Test for pineapple after proteolytic enzymes

1. Symptom-free. Blood sugar 80 milligrams percent. A test meal on the order of 1,225 milligrams of pancreatic enzyme concentrate was given in a powdered pork source.
2. Thirty minutes after step one blood sugar was 80 milligrams percent. Symptom-free. Test meal of pineapple given.
3. One hour after test meal, blood sugar was 130 milligrams percent. Symptom-free.

Results of test: Chemical diabetes was present on the test without proteolytic enzymes. Blood sugar remained normal on test after proteolytic enzymes.

C. Test meal of apple

Test for apple before proteolytic enzymes
Initial reaction: Blood sugar was 200 milligrams percent one hour after the test meal. There were symptoms of nervousness, marked tension, trembling, and anger.

Test for apple after proteolytic enzymes

1. Blood sugar was 80 milligrams percent. Symptom-free. A test meal on the order of 1,670 milligrams pancreatic enzyme concentrate was given in enteric-coated tablets plus glutamic acid HCL, betaine HCL, and pepsin.

2. Thirty minutes after step one the patient was symptom-free. The apple test meal was given.
3. Forty-five minutes after the test meal, blood sugar was 80 milligrams percent. Symptom-free. A quarter of a teaspoon of sodium bicarbonate was given.

Results of test: Test meal of apple without proteolytic enzymes produced diabetic hyperglycemia and marked symptoms. Test meal of apple with proteolytic enzymes produced no symptoms, and blood sugar remained normal.

The following tests are evidence of the fact that proteolytic enzymes plus amino acids can be used to reduce or eliminate cerebral allergic reactions in moderate to severe degenerative disease. As we have seen, deficient proteolytic enzymes lead to a deficiency of essential amino acids. Therefore, amino acids need to be routinely supplemented in pancreatic insufficiency. At the beginning of therapy, amino-acid supplementation is of equal importance to supplementing proteolytic enzymes. Free amino acids can be supplied as capsules, tablets, or predigested protein as liquid-free amino acids. Approximately 15 grams of free amino acids four times a day should be supplied for a minimum of one month and then reduced according to the individual's need.

After one week of proteolytic-enzyme therapy plus amino acids, the following patient had complete relief from reactions to all petrochemical hydrocarbon exposures, whereas before, even while on megavitamins and a diet of avoidance of incriminated foods, he was severely reacting to contact with auto exhaust, perfumes, a gas stove, and so forth.

Schizophrenic—Male: Age 23

Test of sublingual auto exhaust

Test for sublingual auto exhaust before proteolytic enzymes and amino acids

Initial reaction: After the exposure, there were immediate symptoms of marked negativism, loss of insight, loss of motivation, reduced ability to concentrate, reduced comprehension, and painful tension in back and neck.

Test for sublingual auto exhaust after proteolytic enzymes only

1. Five tablets pancreas compound (325 milligrams) plus duodenum. Five tablets bromelain (100 milligrams) plus papain duodenum.
2. Thirty minutes after step one, five tablets pancreas compound plus duodenum and five tablets bromelain plus papain were given.
3. Thirty minutes after step two, the sublingual test for auto exhaust was given.
4. Symptoms: Talkative, spaced-out feeling, poor concentration, difficulty in reading, poor comprehension of what was read, tension, tapping of feet, and headache.

Test for sublingual auto exhaust after proteolytic enzymes plus amino acids

1. Five tablets pancreas compound with duodenum. Five tablets bromelain with papain. Fifteen grams free amino acids!
2. Thirty minutes after step one, five tablets pancreas compound plus duodenum and five tablets bromelain with papain were given. Fifteen grams of free amino acids as predigested protein were also supplied.
3. Thirty minutes after step two, auto exhaust given as a sublingual test.
4. Symptoms: There were no mental symptoms! There was a minor and brief nasal stuffiness at the beginning of the test.

Before enzyme therapy began, this twenty-three-year-old patient violated his rotation diet by eating a meal of Mexican food, and he suffered numerous and very severe mental symptoms. However, one week after enzyme therapy plus amino-acid therapy began, he purposely ate as a test another meal of Mexican food. The startling results were that absolutely no symptoms were experienced.

Examination format for hypo/hyperglycemia

Deliberate Food Testing: There are four days of fasting, with a blood-sugar test each morning. Testing of meals of single foods begins on the fifth day. Blood sugar is taken immediately before each meal and one hour after each meal with more blood-sugar monitoring if desirable. A less accurate method is to test urine sugar prior to and hourly during the test. Three meals a day may be used, and if there are few reactions to foods, then four meals a day may be used. Blood sugar should be normal before each meal, and there should be no sugar in the urine. Each symptom, physical and mental, including an abnormal rise in blood sugar or urine sugar, is evidence of maladaptive reaction to a food.

Inhalant testing: Blood sugar should be monitored before and after each test. Tobacco and petrochemicals are especially prone to evoking hypo/hyperglycemic reactions. Sublingual (under the tongue) and sniff-provocative testing procedures are recommended as appropriate to the specific inhalant substance.

Skin Testing: Intradermal serial-dilution skin testing can serve as a partially effective screening method, but it is less accurate, especially for foods, than deliberate food tests. Again, it may be stated that a rise in blood sugar may be the only symptom evoked by a particular food; this may occur when a skin test otherwise indicates normal.

Treatment format

An individually determined proper diet is the cornerstone of all hypo/hyperglycemia treatment. In order to determine specific nutritional needs in their patients, many orthomolecular physicians run a computerized diet survey. It is a simple computerized test of questions and answers that relate to the individual's entire nutritional-dietary habits. It points out deficiencies of all kinds (i.e., vitamins, minerals, trace elements, bulk and fiber, amino acids, calories, cholesterol, sugar, polyunsaturates, protein-fat-carbohydrates) and gives an accurate nutritional foundation on which to base the treatment of metabolic disorders.

When studying a patient's dietary habits, allergic reactions to specific foods must be taken into consideration. Allergic reactions are dependent to some degree on nutritional and hormonal deficiencies, and metabolic errors in tolerating specific food families. Frequently eaten foods to which a patient is allergic often cause the most severe maladaptive reactions. These reactions are controlled by avoidance of incriminated allergens for three months, followed by reintroduction into a basic four-day food rotation diet. One of the most impressive facts about this is that, based on clinical findings, it has been demonstrated that, after the three-month period in which metabolic normalization is achieved via megavitamin-mineral-amino acid-enzyme-hormone supplementation, a limited infrequent exposure to the incriminating foods will usually not evoke the symptoms previously encountered. After this period of achieving metabolic homeostasis, the patient can often (not always) space his exposure to previously determined food allergens to as frequently as every fourth day, since it takes approximately four days for a single food to be entirely eliminated from the body.

Foods should always be avoided and then rotated every fourth day in families since there may be cross-allergic reactions between family members. For example, tomatoes, potatoes, bell peppers, and tobacco are all of the same food family. If symptoms are evoked by this entire family of foods, then each food within this family should be first avoided for three months and then rotated on a four-day basis. More specifically, this means that if one eats tomatoes on Monday, she should not eat potatoes, bell peppers, or tomatoes until Friday of that same week. It is important to understand that this plan not only reduces allergic-type reactions, but it also increases one's exposure to a greater number of different foods; thus, one's nutritional needs have a better chance of being met by the broader spectrum of nutrients now being encountered. (See page 42 on diversified rotation for other possible formats of rotation.)

A small number of patients have, and a minority of foods are, fixed food allergies. These are easy to diagnose because each time the patient eats the specific allergen, symptoms develop. Chemicals, tobacco, hydrocarbons, coffee, alcohol, sugar, and the grain family often fall into the "fixed allergy" classification and should be avoided if necessary. It is interesting to note that people who react to petrochemical hydrocarbons usually also react to one or more of the certified food colorings. Many prepared foods contain colorings, preservatives, and other substances to which sensitive people can react maladaptively. Even fluoridated water can be a problem.

These clinical observations lead us to the following conclusions: There is an individualized assortment of frequently used foods and chemicals to which a hypoglycemic and diabetic responds maladaptively with physical and emotional symptoms. Each case has to be individually assessed to determine the specific foods or chemicals incriminated for that individual. A glucose-tolerance test used by many physicians today as a single food test (i.e., corn or grape sugar) is inadequate for broad-spectrum judgments in that it reveals the reaction to only one specific food. Accordingly, the generalization that testing one food (corn or grape sugar) is adequate from which to judge all other foods in that same category, such as carbohydrates, can no longer be accepted as true. Clinical food and chemical-induction testing has revealed the surprising evidence that hypo/hyperglycemic reactions to carbohydrates are very selective and not limited strictly to the carbohydrate family. In short, the specificity and individuality of all foods and chemicals need to be recognized and assessed. Any foods, including proteins, fats, and carbohydrates, are possibilities to be incriminated as symptom evokers and hypo/hyperglycemia producers. These specifics of each case will not be known unless individual test meals are performed.

Therefore, it seems valid to conclude that both hypoglycemia and hyperglycemia have the same basic source of allergy-addiction in the majority of cases. Whether the response is low or high blood sugar depends on the stage of the stress reaction. Hypoglycemia can be characterized as the adaptation stage (Hans Selye, *The Stress of Life*) of the stress allergic reaction with the characteristic reaction of hyperinsulinism. Hyperglycemia can be characterized as the exhaustion stage of the stress allergic reaction with the characteristic reaction of hypoinsulinism. The basic treatment is the same for either condition: avoidance and, later, spacing of the individualized symptom-producing foods and chemicals. If this type of ecologic dietary and environmental treatment is not given, the progression of the development from hypoglycemia to adult onset diabetes mellitus is suggested in this order:

1. acute allergic reactions to foods and chemicals, with the allergic reaction first involving the pancreas and/or liver;
2. several years of adaptive addictive adjustment with the consequences of episodic hypoglycemia; and
3. metabolic failure by fatigue and/or exhaustion of the adaptation stage resulting in a degeneration of the pancreas and the logical onset of diabetes mellitus.

The deterioration of various tissues (especially cardiovascular tissues) is best explained as due to the continued, prolonged, and intense stress (i.e., unresolved kinin inflammation in specific tissue targets) caused by numerous foods and chemicals to which a patient is reacting maladaptively. Such a deterioration can likely best be stopped by adequate management of allergies.

However, it would be unfair to say that the proper management of one's diet and chemical environment alone can eliminate the painful symptoms of hypoglycemia and hyperglycemia. Continued allergic stresses on the biochemical system always cause nutritional deficiencies that must be treated with orthomolecular-ecologic methods. These methods include vitamin and mineral supplementation, hormone adjustments, and proteolytic-enzyme and amino-acid therapy.

Any vitamin-mineral supplementation program for hypoglycemia and hyperglycemia must always be tailored to individual biochemical needs. The following daily amounts of vitamins have been suggested for treatment, though these requirements vary greatly among individuals:

Nutrient	***Dosage***
Vitamin C	1 to 4 g three times daily (t.i.d.)
Vitamin A	5,000 to 10,000 IU (t.i.d.)
Vitamin D	100 to 400 IU (t.i.d.)
Vitamin E	100 to 400 IU (t.i.d.)
Vitamin B_1	50 to 500 mg (t.i.d.)
Vitamin B_2	50 to 500 mg (t.i.d.)
Vitamin B_3	250 to 1,000 mg (t.i.d.)
Vitamin B_6	50 to 500 mg (t.i.d.)
Choline	300 mg (t.i.d.)
Inositol	90 mg (t.i.d.)
Bioflavonoids	350 mg (t.i.d.)
Pantothenic acid	50 to 500 mg (t.i.d.)
Folic acid	400 mcg to 5 mg (t.i.d.)
Vitamin B_{15}	50 to 150 mg (t.i.d.)
RNA	400 mg (t.i.d.)
L-Glutamine	50 to 500 mg (t.i.d.)
Hydroxycobalamin	1,000 mcg IM shot (from one shot every two weeks to three shots each week in patients with a deficiency)

Most orthomolecular-ecologic physicians will want to take a hair and/or blood analysis in order to determine the amounts of minerals that are synergistically working with vitamins and other nutrients inside the tissue cell. It is necessary for all the nutritional elements of the cell to be supplied for maximum efficiency and health. It is one thing to eat good food and take a lot of vitamins, but we also need all the essential minerals so that proper absorption and utilization of our other nutrients is accomplished.

The Heidelberg gastrointestinal analysis examination should also be given to all hypo/hyperglycemic patients, since it reveals the presence or absence of normal acid in the stomach as well as the proper bicarbonate production of the pancreas. Both the acid levels and the bicarbonate production are very important because food digestion is dependent on them. Of particular importance is the correct functioning of the pancreas's bicarbonate production. A study by B. M. Frier of adult-onset diabetics revealed a severe reduction in enzymatic and bicarbonate functions of the pancreas.[75] Low enzymatic production by the pancreas has serious consequences. These include reduced digestion of carbohydrates, reduced digestion of fats, and reduced systemic levels of proteolytic enzymes. Proteolytic enzymes digest proteins into amino acids; without adequate proteolytic enzymes, amino-acid deficiencies result. Obviously, a reduced essential-amino-acid supply in the body would also produce many selective nutritional deficiencies (i.e., of vitamins, minerals, hormones), and thus encourage allergic inflammatory reactions to numerous foods and chemicals. Moreover, it is important to realize that small-intestine digestion functions in a neutral to alkaline medium. The pancreas pours out bicarbonate to alkalinize the small intestine. In the hypo/hyperglycemia process, the bicarbonate from the pancreas is reduced, thus further decreasing the efficiency of protein digestion into amino acids. Therefore, it seems logical that in this particular disease process, an external source of bicarbonate should be provided with proteolytic enzymes and amino acids for the intestinal digestive process to occur normally.

These preceding facts have some very interesting implications. In our clinic, we have observed that most hypo/hyperglycemics are capable of the recovery of the pancreas's insulin production if all substances to which the patients are allergically reacting are discovered, avoided, and/or spaced so that all the reactions do not occur. Furthermore, supplementing the proteolytic enzymes and bicarbonate has been observed to aid in normalizing the hormonal production of the pancreas. Thus, a satisfactory treatment regimen requires a discovery of the maladaptive-reacting substances as well as supplementation of pancreatic enzymes, bicarbonate, and, in many cases, amino acids. Only in the most severe cases of diabetes will insulin supplementation be required since insulin production has a better recovery capacity than enzyme and bicarbonate production. This is probably the result of the fact that the islets of Langerhans are the least damaged area of the pancreas when chemical and food maladaptive reactions occur.

Diabetic—age 17

Test meal of pineapple

Test for pineapple before enzymes and amino acids

Initial reaction: Blood sugar was 280 milligrams percent forty minutes after test meal. No subjective or objective symptoms observed.

Test for pineapple after proteolytic enzymes and amino acids

1. Symptom-free. Blood sugar 80 milligrams percent. Fifteen grams of free amino acids and 1,225 milligrams concentrated pancreatic enzymes (pork source) were given.
2. Thirty minutes after step one, blood sugar was still 80 milligrams percent. Symptom-free. Test meal of pineapple given, as well as 1,225 milligrams pancreatic enzymes.
3. Thirty minutes after the test meal, the blood sugar was still 80 milligrams percent. Symptom-free. A quarter of a teaspoon of sodium bicarbonate was given.
4. One hour after test meal, blood sugar was 130 milligrams percent. Symptom-free.

Results of test: Hyperglycemia was present on test without proteolytic enzymes or amino acids. Blood sugar remained normal on test after these substances were given.

Conclusions

Recent observations reveal the hypo/hyperglycemia disease process to involve generalized disordered pancreatic function rather than only selective disordered insulin production. The most seriously curtailed function is that of reduced production of bicarbonate and proteolytic enzymes. We can now understand that the emerging acidosis of the hypo/hyperglycemia reaction is not due only to incomplete metabolism of carbohydrates, lipids, and proteins, but also due to loss of production of bicarbonate by the pancreas. Therefore, we are now prepared to take seriously incomplete indigestion and malabsorption as an aspect of this particular disease process. The far-reaching chain reaction of nutritional and metabolic malfunctions set in motion by this degenerative disease process is staggering to contemplate. No wonder it has been considered a disorder with many and varied complications.

To further clarify the metabolic situation, the following terms and states have been observed as applicable to varying stages of the hypo/hyperglycemia degenerative disease process.

1. Maladaptive kinin and histamine reactions to foods and chemicals.
2. Addiction to certain foods and chemicals.
3. Intestinal malabsorption syndrome and digestive disorders.
4. Deficient proteolytic enzymes and bicarbonate, both at the pancreatic-intestinal level as well as the systemic-cellular level.
5. Acute nutritional deficiencies (i.e., amino acids, vitamins, minerals, and so on), with an essential-amino-acid deficiency as a prominent feature due to the inability of proteolytic enzymes to adequately split amino acids from proteins.
6. Episodic small-intestine acidosis due to decreased pancreatic bicarbonate production.
7. Weakened resistance to infectious invasion.
8. Chronic stress-related breakdown of specific tissue and/or organs.

Understanding these varied states in terms of a degenerative disease process provides a valuable framework for treatment whether its presenting symptomatalogy is mental or physical. See Figure A.1., which pictorially describes the previously discussed contributing factors involved in the pyramid of schizophrenia as well as other mental and emotional disorders.

AUTOIMMUNE REACTION AS MAJOR CAUSE OF SCHIZOPHRENIA

Brain Autoimmune Response Precipitated by
Multiple Opportunist Viral Infections
and Toxins from Microorganisms

VIRAL CANDIDATES

Chronic Remitting Herpes Viruses
Cytomegalovirus
Epstein-Barr virus
Varicella-zoster
Herpes simplex I & II

Enteroviruses
Coxsackieviruses
Echoviruses
Polioviruses

Reoviruses
Influenza/parainfluenza viruses
Rubeola (measles)
Rubella
Unidentified slow viruses
Progenitor cryptocides

METABOLIC DISORDERS/ERRORS
Porphyria
Carnosnuria
Hyperammonemia
Homocystinuria
Toxic methylated amines
Disordered transmethylation
Disordered dophine metabolism
Disordered carbohydrate/insulin metabolism
Genetic predisposition to addictions, especially to foods
Genetic predisposition to allergies, especially to foods
Genetic predisposition to specific infections, especially viral

FOOD ALLERGIES

FOOD ADDICTIONS

CHEMICAL ADDICTIONS
Tobacco
Alcohol
Caffeine
Other drugs

TOXICITIES
Pesticides
Heavy metals
Petrochemicals
Microoganism toxins

OTHER STRESSORS
Physical—
heat, cold
fatigue,
Emotional

NUTRITIONAL DEFICIENCIES | **NUTRITIONAL DEFICIENCIES** | **NUTRITIONAL DEFICIENCIES** | **NUTRITIONAL DEFICIENCIES** | **NUTRITIONAL DEFICIENCIES**

Figure A.1. *Dynamics of the Autoimmune Pyramid in Schizophrenia*

REFERENCES

1. Williams, Roger J., *Nutrition Against Disease* (New York: Pitman, 1971), 11.
2. Fann, William E., "On the Coexistence of Parkinsonism and Tardive Dyskinesia," *Diseases of the Nervous System* 35 (July 1974), 7; Kazamatsuri, H., "Therapeutic Approaches to Tardive Dyskinesia," *Archives of General Psychiatry* 27 (October 1972): 4.
3. Hughes, Harold E., then United States senator, quoted by the Huxley Institute for Biosocial Research, 1114 First Avenue, New York, N.Y. 10021.
4. Hearing before the Select Committee on Nutrition on Human Needs of the United States Senate, June 22, 1977.
5. Rinkel, H. J., T. G. Randolph, and M. Zeller, *Food Allergy* (Springfield, Ill.: Thomas, 1951), 102.
6. Rinkel, *Food Allergy*, 102.
7. Speer, G., *Allergy of the Nervous System* (Springfield, Ill.: Thomas, 1970).
8. Alvarez, W. C., *The Neuroses* (Philadelphia: Saunders, 1952), 42.
9. Speer, *Allergy of the Nervous System*, 63.
10. Alvarez, *The Neuroses*, 466.
11. Rapaport, H. G., *The Complete Allergy Guide* (New York: Simon & Schuster, 1970), 153.
12. Personal unpublished account written by a former patient of Dr. Philpott.
13. Philpott, W. H., R. Nielsen, and V. Pierson, "Four-Day Rotation of Foods According to Families," *Clinical Ecology*, ed. L. D. Dickey (Springfield, Ill.: Thomas, 1976), 474–86.
14. Pritikin, N., *Pritikin Diet and Exercise Program* (New York: Grosset & Dunlap, 1979).
15. Randolph, T. G., "The Descriptive Features of Food Addiction: Addictive Eating and Drinking," *Quarterly Journal for the Study of Alcohol* 17 (1956): 198.

16. Rinkel, *Food Allergy.*
17. Campbell, M. B., "Neurologic Manifestations of Allergic Disease," *Annals of Allergy* 31 (1973).
18. Personal unpublished account written by M. A. Stream, M.D.
19. Pauling, Linus, "Varying the Concentration of Substances Normally Found in the Human Body," *Science* 160 (1968): 265.
20. Williams, Roger J., *Nutrition Against Disease* (New York: Pitman, 1971); Bruno, M., "There's a Psychotherapy in the B Vitamins," *Prevention* 25, no. 4 (1973): 75.
21. Joliffe, N., "Effects of Vitamin Deficiency in Mental and Emotional Process," *Research of Nervous and Mental Disease* 19 (1939): 144; Frostig and Spies, "The Initial Syndrome of Pellagra and Associated Deficiency Diseases," *American Journal of Medical Science* 199 (1940): 268; Hoffer, Abram, Correspondence, *Canadian Medical Association Journal* 109 (1973): 574.
22. Irvine, D. G., "Kryptopyrrole Molecular Psychiatry," *Orthomolecular Psychiatry* (San Francisco: W. H. Freeman, 1973).
23. Newbold, H. L., *Mega-Nutrients for Your Nerves* (New York: Peter H. Wyden, 1975).
24. Williams, *Nutrition Against Disease.*
25. Pfeiffer, C. C., "Blood Histamine, Basophil Counts, and Trace Elements in the Schizophrenias," *Orthomolecular Psychiatry* (San Francisco: Freeman, 1973).
26. Horwitt, M. K., "Ascorbic Acid Requirements of Individuals in a Large Institution," *Proceedings of the Society for Experimental Biology and Medicine* 49 (1942): 248–50.
27. Milner, G., "Ascorbic Acid in Chronic Psychiatric Patients," *British Journal of Psychiatry* 109 (1963): 299.
28. Pauling, Linus, "Results of a Loading Test of Ascorbic Acid," *Journal of Orthomolecular Psychiatry* (1973), 18–34.
29. Black, D. R., "Experimental Potassium Depletion in Man," *Lancet* 1 (1952): 244; Wormsley, G. H., "Potassium and Sodium Restriction in the Normal Human," *Journal of Clinical Investigations* 34 (1955): 456.

30. Williams, R. J., and D. K. Kalita, *A Physician's Handbook on Orthomolecular Medicine* (Los Angeles: Keats, 1979), 78.
31. Reich, C. J., "The Vitamin Therapy of Chronic Asthma," *Journal of Asthma Research* 9 (1971): 32.
32. Arneson, G. A., "Phenothiazine Derivatives and Glucose Metabolism," *Journal of Neuropsychiatry* 5 (1964): 181–85; Hiles, B. W., "Hyperglycemia and Glycasuria Following Chlorpromazine Therapy," *Journal of the American Medical Association* 162 (1956): 165; Norman, D., "Glycemic Effects of Chlorpromazine in the Mouse, Hamster, and Rat, *Proceedings of the Society for Experimental Biology Medicine* 90 (1955): 89–91; Thonnard, N. E., "Phenothiazines and Diabetes in Hospitalized Women," *American Journal of Psychiatry* 124 (1968): 978–82; Waitzkin, "A Survey of Unknown Diabetics in a Mental Hospital," *Diabetes* 15 (1966): 97–104; Zumoff, B., "Aggravation of Diabetic Hyperglycemia by Chlacodiazepoxide," *Journal of the American Medical Association* 237, no. 18, 1977.
33. Williams and Kalita, *A Physician's Handbook on Orthomolecular Medicine*, 2.
34. Ibid., 2.
35. Ibid., 76.
36. Ibid., 46.
37. Ibid., 46.
38. *Executive Health* 12, no. 3, 1975.
39. Stone, I., *The Healing Factor* (New York: Grosset & Dunlap, 1972).
40. *The Linus Pauling Newsletter* 1 (Fall 1978): 4.
41. Ibid.
42. Williams and Kalita, *A Physician's Handbook on Orthomolecular Medicine*, 52.
43. Pauling, Linus, *Vitamin C and the Common Cold* (San Francisco: Freeman, 1976), 115–18.
44. *The Linus Pauling Newsletter*, 4.
45. Strauss, L. H., and P. Scheer, "Effect of Nicotine on Vitamin C

Metabolism," *International Zeitschift fur Vitaminforschung* 9 (1939): 39–48; McCormick, W. J., "Ascorbic Acid As a Chemotherapeutic Agent," *Archives Pediatrics* 69 (1952): 151–55; Bourquin, A. and E. Musmanno, "Effect of Smoking on the Ascorbic Acid Content of Whole Blood," *American Journal of Digestive Diseases* 20 (1953): 75–77; Goyanna, C., "Tobacco and Vitamin C," *Brasil Medico* 69 (1955): 173–77; Calder, J. H. and R. C. Curtis, "Comparison of the Vitamin C in Plasma and Leukocytes of Smokers and Nonsmokers," *Lancet* 1 (1963): 556.

46. Mavin, J. V. "Experimental Treatment of Acute Mercury Poisoning of Guinea Pigs and Ascorbic Acid," *Revista de la Sociedad Argentina de Biologia* 17 (1941): 581–86; Robinson, S. W., "Effect of Vitamin C and Workers Exposed to Lead Dust," *Journal of Laboratory and Clinical Medicine* 26 (1941): 1478–81; Dannenberg, A. M., "Ascorbic Acid in the Treatment of Chronic Lead Poisoning," *Journal of the American Medical Association* 114 (1940): 1439–40; Han-Wen, H., "Treatment of Lead Poisoning: Experiments on the Effect of Vitamin C and Rutin," *Chinese Journal on Internal Medicine* 7 (1959): 19–20.
47. Holmes, H. N., "Effect of Vitamin C on Lead Poisoning," *Journal of Laboratory and Clinical Medicine* 24 (1939): 1119–27.
48. Mokranjac, M. and C. Petrovic, "Vitamin C As an Antidote in Poisoning by Fatal Doses of Mercury," *Comptes Rendus Hebdomadaires des Seances de l'Academie des Sciences* 258 (1964): 1341–42.
49. Milner, G. "Ascorbic Acid in Chronic Psychiatric Patients: A Controlled Trial," *British Journal of Psychiatry* 109 (1963): 294–99.
50. Pauling, Linus, "Results of a Loading Test of Ascorbic Acid," *Journal of Orthomolecular Psychiatry* (1973), 18–34.
51. Newbold, H. L., *Vitamin C Against Cancer* (New York: Stein and Day, 1979), 295–98.
52. *The Linus Pauling Newsletter* 1, no. 4 (Fall 1978).
53. Burton, B. T., ed., *The Heinz Handbook of Nutrition* (New York: McGraw-Hill, 1959).

54. Williams and Kalita, *A Physician's Handbook on Orthomolecular Medicine*, 7.
55. Pauling, *Journal of Orthomolecular Psychiatry* 7, no. 1: 3, 4.
56. Personal conversation between Dr. Hoffer and Dr. Philpott.
57. Selye, Hans, *The Stress of Life* (New York: McGraw Hill, 1956).
58. Potts, John, "Avoidance Provocative Food Testing in Assessing Diabetes Responsiveness," *Diabetes* (1977), 26.
59. Nittler, Alan, "Hypoglycemia and the New Breed of Patient," *Journal of the International Academy of Metabology* 5, no. 1.
60. Williams and Kalita, *A Physician's Handbook on Orthomolecular Medicine*, 157.
61. Seyle, *The Stress of Life.*
62. Tintera, J. W., "Endocrine Aspects of Schizophrenia: Hypoglycemia of Hypoadrenocorticism," *Journal of Schizophrenia* 1 (1967): 150; Tintera, J. W., "The Hypoadrenocortical State and Its Management," *New York State Journal of Medicine* 55 (1955): 1869; Tintera, J. W., "Stabilizing Homeostasis in the Recovered Alcoholic Through Endocrine Therapy: Evaluation of the Hypoglycemia Factor," *Journal of the American Geriatric Society* 14 (1966): 126.
63. Pauling, *Journal of Orthomolecular Psychiatry* 6, no. 2: 187–90.
64. Crane, G. E., "Clinical Psychopharmacology in Its Twentieth Year," *Science* 181 (1973): 124.
65. Asnis, G. M., "A Survey of Tardive Dyskinesia in Psychiatric Outpatients," *American Journal of Psychiatry* 134 (December 1977): 12.
66. Pauling, *Journal of Orthomolecular Psychiatry* 5, no. 1: 5.
67. "Tardive Dyskinesia Associated with Antipsychotic Drugs," *FDA Drug Bulletin* (May 1973).
68. Pauling, *Journal of Orthomolecular Psychiatry* 5, no. 1: 5.
69. Ibid., 6–8.
70. Ibid.
71. Growdon, J. H., "Oral Choline Administration to Patients with Tardive Dyskinesia," *New England Journal of Medicine* 297 (September 1977): 524–27.

72. DeVeaugh-Geiss, J., "High-Dose Pyridoxine in Tardive Dyskinesia," *Journal of Clinical Psychiatry* 39, no. 6 (June 1978).
73. Personal unpublished account written by Donna M. Calvera.
74. Robertson, E. A., A. C. Van Steirteghem, J. E. Byrkit, and D. S. Young, *Clinical Chemistry* 26, no. 1 (1980): 30–36.
75. Frier, B. M., "Exocrine Pancreatic Function in Juvenile-Onset Diabetes Mellitus," *Gut* 17 (1976): 685–91.

SUGGESTED READING

Adams, R. and F. Murray. *Megavitamin Therapy.* New York: Larchmont, 1973.

Altschule, M. D. and Z. L. Hegedus. "The Adrenochrome Hypothesis of Schizophrenia," originally published in 1972; "The Role of Rheomelanin Formation in Some Toxic Effects of Catecholamine Derivatives." In *Orthomolecular Psychiatry, Treatment of Schizophrenia,* edited by D. Hawkins and L. Pauling. San Francisco: Freeman, 1973.

Altschul, R. *Niacin in Vascular Disorders and Hyperlipemia.* Springfield, Ill.: Thomas, 1964.

Angel, C., B. E. Leach, S. Martens, M. Cohen, and R. G. Health. "Serum Oxidation Levels." *Archives of Neurological Psychiatry* 78 (1957): 500.

Aring, C. D., J. P. Evans, and T. D. Spies. "Some Clinical Neurologic Aspects of Vitamin B Deficiencies." *Journal of American Medical Association* 113 (1939): 2105.

Aring, C. D. and T. D. Spies. "A Critical Review: Vitamin B Deficiency and Nervous Disease." *Journal of Neurological Psychiatry* 2 (1939): 335.

Axelrod, A. E. and A. C. Trakatellis. "Relationship of Pyridoxine to Immunological Phenomena." *Vitamins and Hormones* 22 (1964): 59.

Baker, E. M. "Ascorbic Acid Metabolism in Man." *American Journal of Clinical Nutrition* 19 (1967): 583.

Bicknell, F. and F. Prescott. *The Vitamin in Medicine.* Milwaukee: Lee Foundation, 1953.

Black, D. A. K. "Experimental Potassium Depletion in Man." *Lancet* 1 (1952): 244.

Blackman, D., S. Blackman, A. Thomason, and N. Thomason. "The Blackman-Thomason Salts Technique for Treating Opiate Addiction." Berkeley, 1973.

Brin, M. *Newer Methods of Nutritional Biochemistry.* New York: Academic Press, 1967.

Brozek, J. "Nutritional Research in the Soviet Union: I. Some General Aspects." *Nutrition Reviews* 19 (1961): 129–32.

———. "Nutritional Research in the Soviet Union: II. Some Specific Aspects." *Nutrition Reviews* 19 (1961): 161–64.

Bruno, M. "There's Psychotherapy in the B Vitamins." *Prevention* 25, no. 4 (1973): 75.

Buckley, R. E. "Hypothalamic Tuning, Hypoglycemia Episodes and Schizophrenic Responses." *Schizophrenia* 1 (1969): 1.

Burton, R. M., R. Salvador, K. Smith, and R. E. Howard. "The Effect of Chlorpromazine, Nicotinamide and Nicotinic Acid on Pyridine Nucleotide Levels of Human Blood." *Annals of the New York Academy of Science* 96 (1962): 195.

Campbell, M. B. "Allergy and Behavior: Neurologic and Psychic Syndromes." In *Allergy of the Nervous System,* edited by F. Speer. Springfield, Ill.: Thomas, 1970.

Careddu, P., L. T. Tenconi, and G. Sacchetti. "Transmethylation in Mongols." *Lancet* 1 (1963): 828.

Carter, C. H. *Handbook of Mental Retardation Syndromes.* Springfield, Ill.: Thomas, 1970.

Cheraskin, E. and W. M. Ringsdorf. *New Hope for Incurable Diseases.* New York: Exposition Press, 1971.

Cohen, G. and P. Hochstein. "Enzymatic Mechanisms of Drug Sensitivity in the Brain." *Diseases of the Nervous System* 24 (1963): 44.

Conney, A. H., G. A. Bray, C. Evans, and J. J. Burns. "Metabolic Interactions Between L-Ascorbic Acid and Drugs." *Annals of the New York Academy of Science* 92 (1961): 115.

Cordas, S. Personal Correspondence, Eulis, Texas, 1975.

Cott, A. "Treating Schizophrenic Children." *Schizophrenia* 1 (1967): 3.

———. "Continued Fasting Treatment of Schizophrenics in the U.S.S.R." *Schizophrenia* 1 (1969): 44.

———. *Orthomolecular Treatment: A Biochemical Approach to Treatment of Schizophrenia.* New York: Huxley Insitute for Biosocial Research, 1970.

———. "Megavitamins: The Orthomolecular Approach to Behavioral Approach to Behavioral Disorders and Learning Disabilities." *Journal of Schizophrenia* 3 (1971): 1.

———. "Megavitamins: The Orthomolecular Approach to Behavioral Approach to Behavioral Disorders and Learning Disabilities." *Academic Therapy* 7 (1972): 245.

Davis, S. D., T. Nelson, and T. H. Shepard. "Teratogenecity of Vitamin B_6 Deficiency: Omphalocele, Skeletal and Neural Defects, and Splenic Hypoplasia." *Science* 196 (1970): 1329.

Davis, V. E. and M. J. Walsh. "Alcohol, Amines, and Alkaloids: A Possible Biochemical Basis for Alcohol Addiction." *Science* 167 (1970): 3920.

Dayton, P. G. and N. Weiner. "Ascorbic Acid and Blood Coagulation." *Annals of New York Academy of Science* 92 (1961): 302.

Dohan, F. C. "Is Celiac Disease A Clue to the Pathogenesis of Schizophrenia?" *Mental Hygiene* 53 (1969): 4.

Dohan, F. C., J. C. Grasberger, F. M. Lowell, H. T. Johnston, and A. W. Abbegast. "Relapsed Schizophrenics: More Rapid Improvement on a Milk and Cereal Free Diet." *British Journal of Psychiatry* 115 (1969): 522.

Eiduson, G., E. Geller, A. Yuwiler, and B. T. Eiduson. *Biochemistry and Behavior*. Princeton: Van Nostrand, 1964.

Ellis, J. M. *Vitamin B_6: The Doctor's Report*. New York: Harper & Row, 1973.

El Meligi, A. M. and H. Osmond. "The Experiential World Inventory in Clinical Psychiatry and Psychopharmacology." In *Orthomolecular Psychiatry, Treatment of Schizophrenia,* edited by D. Hawkins and L. Pauling. San Francisco: Freeman, 1973.

Ferstrom, J. D. and R. J. Wurtman. "Brain Serotonin Content: Increase Following Ingestion of Carbohydrate Diet." *Science* 174 (1971): 1028.

Fogel, S. and A. Hoffer. "The Use of Hypnosis to Interpret and to Reproduce an LSD-25 Experience." *Journal of Clinical and Experimental Psychopathology* 23 (1962): 44.

Fredericks, C. *Eating Right for You*. New York: Grosset & Dunlap, 1972.

———. "Hotline to Health." *Prevention* 26, no. 10 (1974): 59.

Frostig, J. P. and T. D. Spies. "The Initial Syndrome of Pellagra and Associated Deficiency Diseases." *American Journal of Medical Science* 199 (1940): 268.

Gillman, J., and T. Gillman. *Perspectives in Human Malnutrition.* New York: Grune and Stratton, 1951.

Golden, R. L., R. S. Mortati, and G. A. Schroeter. Correspondence. *Journal of the American Medical Association* 213 (1970): 628.

Goldstein, L. and R. A. Beck. "Amplitude Analyses of the Electroencephalogram." *International Reviews of Neurobiology* 8 (1965): 125.

Goodhart, R. S. "The Role of Nutritional Factors in the Cause, Prevention and Cure of Alcoholism and Associated Infirmities." *American Journal of Clinical Nutrition* 5 (1957): 612.

Gordon, G. S., F. M. Estess, J. E. Adams, K. M. Bowman, and A. Simon. "Cerebral Oxygen Uptake in Chronic Schizophrenia Reactions." *Archives of Neurological Psychiatry* 73 (1955): 544.

Gottlieb, J. S., C. E. Frohman, and C. R. Harmison. "Schizophrenia: New Concepts." *Southern Medical Journal* 64 (1971): 743.

Grant, D. *Recipe for Survival.* Los Angeles: Keats, 1974.

Green, R. G. Correspondence. *Canadian Medical Association Journal* 100 (1969): 586.

———. Correspondence. *Canadian Medical Association Journal* 110 (1974): 617.

Greenberg, S. M. "Iron Absorption and Metabolism." *Journal of Nutrition* 63 (1957): 19.

Gullino, P., M. Winitz, S. M. Birnbaum, J. Cornfield, M. C. Otey, and J. P. Grunstein. "Studies on the Metabolism of Amino Acids and Related Compounds in Vitro." *Archives of Internal Medicine* 128 (1971): 596.

Hart, R. J. "Psychosis in Vitamin B_{12} Deficiency." *Archives of Internal Medicine* 128 (1971): 596.

Hawkins, D. R. "Treatment of Schizophrenia." *Journal of Schizophrenia* 2 (1968): 3.

———. "IV. A Practical Clinical Model." In *Orthomolecular Psychiatry, Treatment of Schizophrenia*, edited by D. Hawkins and L. Pauling. San Francisco: Freeman, 1973.

Heath, R. G. "Schizophrenia: Biochemical and Physiologic Aberrations." *International Journal of Neuropsychiatry* 2 (1966): 597.

Herbert, V. "A Palatable Diet for Producing Experimental Folate Deficiency in Man." *American Journal of Clinical Nutrition* 12 (1963): 17.

Herjanic, M. "Ascorbic Acid and Schizophrenia." In *Orthomolecular Psychiatry, Treatment of Schizophrenia*, edited by D. Hawkins and L. Pauling. San Francisco: Freeman, 1973.

Himwich, H. E. *Brain Metabolism and Cerebral Disorders*. Baltimore: Williams & Wilkins, 1951.

Hoffer, A. *Niacin Therapy in Psychiatry*. Springfield, Ill.: Thomas, 1962.

———. Correspondence. *Canadian Medical Association Journal* 107 (1972): 112.

———. Correspondence. *Canadian Medical Association Journal* 109 (1973): 574.

———. "Mechanism of Action of Nicotinic Acid and Nicotinamide in the Treatment of Schizophrenia." In *Orthomolecular Psychiatry, Treatment of Schizophrenia*, edited by D. Hawkins and L. Pauling. San Francisco: Freeman, 1973.

Hoffer, A. and H. Osmond. "Double-Blind Clinical Trials." *Journal of Neuropsychiatry* 2 (1961): 221.

———. "In reply." *Journal of Neuropsychiatry* 3 (1961): 262.

———. *The Chemical Basis of Clinical Psychiatry*. Springfield, Ill.: Thomas, 1962.

———. "Some Psychological Consequences of Perceptual Disorders in Schizophrenia." *International Journal of Neuropsychiatry* 2 (1966): 1.

Hoffer, A. and M. Walker. *Nutrients to Age Without Senility*. Los Angeles: Keats, 1980.

———. *Orthomolecular Nutrition*. Los Angeles: Keats, 1978.

Horwitt, M. K., B. J. Meyer, A. C. Meyer, C. C. Harvey, and D. Haffron. "Serum Copper and Oxidase Activity in Schizophrenia Patterns." *Archives of Neurology and Psychiatry* 78 (1957): 275.

Hurley, L. S. "Zinc Deficiency in the Developing Rat." *American Journal of Clinical Nutrition* 22 (1969): 1332.

Huxley, J. "Evolution: The Modern Synthesis." *Heredity* 9 (1964): 1.

Irvine, D. G. "Kryptopyrrole in Molecular Psychiatry." In *Orthomolecular Psychiatry, Treatment of Schizophrenia*, edited by D. Hawkins and L. Pauling. San Francisco: Freeman, 1973.

Joliffe, N. "Effects of Vitamin Deficiency on Mental and Emotional Processes." *Research of Nervous and Mental Disease* 19 (1939): 144.

Joliffe, N., K. M. Bowman, L. A. Roseblum, and H. D. Fein. "Nicotonic Acid Deficiency Encephalopathy." *Journal of the American Medical Association* 114 (1940): 307.

Josephson, E. *Thymus, Manganese, and Myasthenia Gravis.* New York: Chedney, 1961.

Karlsson, J. L. *The Biological Basis of Schizophrenia.* Springfield, Ill.: Thomas, 1966.

Kelm, H. "An Evaluation of the Hoffer-Osmond Diagnostic Test." *Journal of Schizophrenia* 1 (1967): 90.

Kety, S. S., R. B. Woodford, M. Harmel, F. A. Freyhan, K. E. Appel, and C. F. Schmidt. "Cerebral Blood Flow and Metabolism in Schizophrenia." *American Journal of Psychiatry* 104 (1948): 765.

Kittler, F. J. "The Effect of Allergy on Children with Minimal Brain Damage." In *Allergy of the Nervous System*, edited by R. Speer. Springfield, Ill.: Thomas, 1970.

Klenner, F. R. "Virus Pneumonia and Its Treatment with Vitamin C." *Southern Medical Surgery* (February 1948).

———. "Massive Doses of Vitamin C and the Virus Diseases." *Southern Medical Surgery* (1951).

———. "The Treatment of Trichinosis with Massive Doses of Vitamin C and Para-Aminobenzoic Acid." *Tri-State Medical Journal* (1952).

———. "The Role of Ascorbic Acid in Therapeutics." *Tri-State Medical Journal* (November 1955).

———. "A New Office Procedure for the Determination of Plasma Levels for Ascorbic Acid." *Tri-State Medical Journal* 5 (1956).

———. "An Insidious Virus." *Tri-State Medical Journal* (June 1957).

———. "Encephalitis as a Sequelae of the Pneumonias." *Tri-State Medical Journal* (February 1960).

Knox, W. E. "An Evaluation of the Treatment of Phenylketonuria with Diets Low in Phenylalanine." *Pediatrics* 26 (1960): 1.

Kornetsky, C. and A. Mirsky. "On Certain Pharmacological and Physiological Differences Between Schizophrenics and Normal Persons." *Psychopharmacology* 8 (1966): 309.

Kowalson, B. "Metabolic Dysperception: The Role of the Family Physician in Its Diagnosis and Management." In *Orthomolecular Psychiatry, Treatment of Schizophrenia*, edited by D. Hawkins and L. Pauling. San Francisco: Freeman, 1973.

Krippner, S. "Illicit Drug Usage: Hazards for Learning Disabled Students." *Orthomolecular Psychiatry* 1 (1972): 1.

LeClair, E. R. "A Report on the Use of Orthomolecular Therapy in a California State Hospital." *Orthomolecular Psychiatry* 1 (1972): 2–3.

Lewis, W. W. "Continuity and Intervention in Emotional Disturbance: A Review." *Exceptional Children* 31 (1965): 467.

Lieber, C. S. and L. M. DeCarli. "Reduced Nicotinamide Adenine Dinucleotide Phosphate Oxidase: Activity Enhanced by Ethanol Consumption." *Science* 170 (1970): 3953.

Lilliston, L. "The Megavitamin Controversy." *Los Angeles Times*, November 26, 1972.

Lucas, A. R., K. Warner, and J. S. Gottlieb. "Biological Studies in Childhood Schizophrenia: Serotonin Uptake by Platelets." *Biological Psychiatry* 3 (1971): 123.

Ludeman, K. and L. Henderson. *The Do-It-Yourself Allergy Analysis Handbook*. Los Angeles: Keats, 1979.

Maas, J. W., G. C. Gleser, and L. A. Gottschalk. "Schizophrenia Anxiety, and Biochemical Factors." *Archives of General Psychiatry* 4 (1961): 109.

Mandell, M. "May Emotional Reactions Be Precipitated by Allergens?" *Connecticut Medicine* 32 (1968).

———. "Cerebral Manifestations of Hypersensitivity to the Chemical Environment: Susceptibility to Indoor and Outdoor Pollution." *Review Allergy* 22 (1968).

———. "Cerebral Reactions in Allergic Patients." New England Foundation for Allergic and Environmental Diseases. Norwalk, Connecticut, 1969.

———. "Allergies Alleged to be the Cause of Psychosis." New England Foundation for Allergic and Environmental Diseases. Norwalk, Connecticut, January 1970.

———. "Central Nervous System Hypersensitivity to House Dust, Molds, and Foods." *Review Allergy* 24 (1970).

Martin, G. R. "Studies on the Tissue Distribution of Ascorbic Acid." *Annals of the New York Academy of Science* 92 (1961): 141.

Martin, P. "Mentally Ill Children Respond to Nutrition." *Prevention* 26, no. 2 (1974): 95.

Mason, A. S. "Endocrine and Metabolic Disorders." *British Journal of Clinical Practice* 12 (1958): 732.

Mayer, J. "Chromium in Medicine." *Postgraduate Medicine* 49 (1971): 235.

———. *Human Nutrition.* Springfield, Ill.: Thomas, 1972.

McGrath, S. D., P. F. O'Brien, P. J. Power, and J. R. Shea. "Megavitamin Treatment of Schizophrenia." *Schizophrenia Bulletin* 5 (1972): 74.

Meiers, R. L. "Relative Hypoglycemia in Schizophrenia." In *Orthomolecular Psychiatry, Treatment of Schizophrenia,* edited by D. Hawkins and L. Pauling. San Francisco: Freeman, 1973.

Millar, J. A., A. Goldberg, and S. Hernberg. "Lead and Delta-Aminolevulinic Acid Dehydratase Levels in Mentally Retarded Children and in Lead-Poisoned Suckling Rats." *Lancet* 2 (1970): 695.

Milner, G. "Ascorbic Acid in Chronic Schizophrenia Patients: A Controlled Test." *British Journal of Psychiatry* 109 (1963): 294.

Moncrieff, A. A. "Lead Poisoning in Children." *Archives of Diseases in Children* 39 (1964): 1

Newbold, H. L. *Mega-Nutrients for Your Nerves.* New York: Peter H. Wyden Publisher, 1975, 65–69.

Nicolson, G. A., A. D. Greiner, W. J. McFarlane, and R. A. Baker. "Effects of Penicillamine on Schizophrenic Patients." *Lancet* 2 (1966): 344.

Olson, R. E., D. Gursey, and J. W. Vester. "Evidence for a Defect in Tryptophan Metabolism in Chronic Alcoholism." *New England Journal of Medicine* 263 (1960): 1169.

Osmond, H. and A. Hoffer. "A Comprehensive Theory of Schizophrenia." *International Journal of Neuropsychiatry* 2 (1966): 303.

Papez, J. W. "Form of Living Organisms in Psychotic Patients." *Journal of Nervous and Mental Disease* 116 (1952): 375.

———. "The Hypophysis Cerebric in Psychosis." *Journal of Nervous and Mental Disease* 119 (1954): 326.

Pauling, L. "Orthomolecular Psychiatry: Varying the Concentrations of Substances Normally Present in the Human Body May Control Mental Disease." *Science* 160 (1968): 265.

———. *Vitamin C and the Common Cold.* San Francisco: Freeman, 1970.

———. "Orthomolecular Psychiatry." In *Orthomolecular Psychiatry, Treatment of Schizophrenia*, edited by D. Hawkins and L. Pauling. San Francisco: Freeman, 1973.

Perry, T. L., S. Hansen, B. Tischler, R. Bonting, and S. Diamond. "Glutamine Depletion in Phenylketonuria." *New England Journal of Medicine* 282 (1970): 761.

Pfeiffer, C. C., V. Iliev, and L. Goldstein. "Blood Histamine, Basophil Counts, and Trace Elements in the Schizophrenias." In *Orthomolecular Psychiatry, Treatment of Schizophrenia*, edited by D. Hawkins and L. Pauling. San Francisco: Freeman, 1973.

Philpott, W. H. "Ecologic and Supernutrition Methods of Determining Values of Orthomolecular Psychiatry Treatment." November 1973.

———. "Methods of Relief of Acute and Chronic Symptoms of Deficiency-Allergy-Addiction Maladaptive Reactions to Foods and Chemicals." Paper presented at the meeting of Seventh Advanced Seminar in Clinical Ecology, Fort Lauderdale, Florida, January 9, 1974.

Portis, S. A. "Emotions and Hyperinsulinism." *Journal of the American Medical Association* 142 (1950): 1291.

Powers, H. W. S. "Dietary Measures to Improve Behavior and Achievement." *Academic Therapy* 9 (1973): 3.

Randolph, T. G. "Allergic Factors in the Etiology of Certain Mental Symptoms." *Journal of Laboratory and Clinical Medicine* 36 (December 1950): 977.

———. "Sensitivity to Petroleum: Including Its Derivatives and Antecedents." *Journal of Laboratory and Clinical Medicine* 40 (December 1952): 931–32.

———. "Depressions Caused by Home Exposures to Gas and Combustion Products of Gas, Oil and Coal." *Journal of Laboratory and Clinical Medicine* 46 (December 1955): 942.

———. "Specific Adaptation Syndrome." *Journal Laboratory & Clinical Medicine* 48 (December 1956): 934.

———. "Ecologic Mental Illness—Psychiatry Exteriorized." *Journal of Laboratory and Clinical Medicine* 54 (December 1959): 936.

———. "A Third Dimension of the Medical Investigation." *Clinical Physiology* 2 (Winter 1960): 1–5.

———. "Ecologic Mental Illness—Levels of Central Nervous System Reactions." Proceedings of the Third World Congress of Psychiatry, vol. 1, Montreal, Canada, University of Toronto Press (June 1961): 379–84.

———. *Human Ecology and Susceptibility to the Chemical Environment.* Springfield, Ill.: Thomas, 1962.

———. "Man-Made Seasonal Sickness." *Journal of Laboratory and Clinical Medicine* 62 (1963): 1005–6.

———. *Proceedings of the National Conference on Air Pollution.* U.S. Department of Health, Education and Welfare. Public Health Service Publication No. 1022. Washington, D.C.: U.S. Government Printing Office 157 (1963).

———. "The Ecologic Unit." *Hospital Management* 97 (March 1964): 45–47; (April 1964): 46–48.

———. "The Provocative Hydrocarbon Test, Preliminary Report." *Journal of Laboratory and Clinical Medicine* 64 (December 1964): 995.

———. "An Ecologic Orientation in Medicine: Comprehensive Environmental Control in Diagnosis and Therapy." *Annals of Allergy* 23 (1965): 7–22.

———. "Clinical Ecology As It Affects the Psychiatric Patient." *International Journal of Social Psychiatry* 12 (Autumn 1966): 245–54.

———. "Stimulatory and Withdrawal Phases and Levels of Chronically Occurring and Experimentally Induced Ecologic Mental Disturbances." Program, 2d International Congress of Social Psychiatry, August 1969. Submitted for publication.

———. "The Role of Specific Adaptation in Chronic Illness." Submitted for publication.

Rapaport, H. G. "Chronic Illness." *Annals of Allergy* 26 (1968): 230–32.

Ridges, A. P. "The Methylation Hypothesis in Relation to 'Pink Spot' and Other Investigations." In *Orthomolecular Psychiatry, Treatment of Schizophrenia*, edited by D. Hawkins and L. Pauling. San Francisco: Freeman, 1973.

Rimland, B. *Infantile Autism: the Syndrome and Its Implications for a Neural Theory of Behavior.* New York: Appleton-Century-Crofts, 1964.

———. *High-Dosage Levels of Certain Vitamins in the Treatment of Children with Severe Mental Disorders.* San Diego: Institute for Child Behavior Research, 1968.

———. "High-Dosage Levels of Certain Vitamins in the Treatment of Children with Severe Mental Disorders." In *Orthomolecular Psychiatry, Treatment of Schizophrenia*, edited by D. Hawkins and L. Pauling. San Francisco: Freeman, 1973.

Rinkel, H. J., T. G. Randolph, and M. Zeller. *Food Allergy.* Springfield, Ill.: Thomas, 1951.

Robie, T. R. "A Review of Ten Years' Experience Utilizing Niacin in Treating Schizophrenia with an Evaluation of Metabolic Dysperception as a Clarifying Diagnostic Term." In *Orthomolecular Psychiatry, Treatment of Schizophrenia*, edited by D. Hawkins and L. Pauling. San Francisco: Freeman, 1973.

Rodale, R. "The Zinc Story." *Prevention* 25, no. 7 (1973): 21.

———. "Putting More Zinc into Your Life." *Prevention* 25, no. 8 (1973): 21.

———. "You Can Solve Your Zinc Problem." *Prevention* 25, no. 9 (1973): 21.

———. "Creeping Vegetarianism Creates Zinc Hunger." *Prevention* 26, no. 7 (1974): 21.

Rosenberg, L. E. "Vitamin-Dependent Genetic Disease." *Hospital Practice* (1970): 59.

Scheid, A. S. "Comparison of Methods for Determination of Vitamin B_{12} Potency." *Journal of Nutrition* 47 (1952): 601.

Schroeder, H. A. *The Trace Elements and Man*. Old Greenwich, Conn.: Devin-Adair, 1973.

———. *The Poisons Around Us*. Los Angeles: Keats, 1978.

Shils, M. E. "Experimental Human Magnesium Depletion." *American Journal of Clinical Nutrition* 15 (1964): 133.

Speer, E., ed. *Allergy of the Nervous System*. Springfield, Ill.: Thomas, 1970.

Stone, I. *The Healing Factor: Vitamin C Against Disease*. New York: Grosset & Dunlap, 1972.

Tui, C. O. "The Fundamentals of Clinical Proteinology." *Journal of Clinical Nutrition* 1 (1953): 232.

Turkel, H. *New Hope for the Mentally Retarded*. New York: Vantage, 1972.

Urbach, C., K. Hickman, and P. L. Harris. "Effect of Individual Vitamins A, C, and E and Carotene Administered at High Levels on Their Concentration in the Blood." *Experimental Surgery* 10 (1952): 7.

Vanderkamp, A. "A Biochemical Abnormality in Schizophrenia Involving Ascorbic Acid." *International Journal of Neuropsychiatry* 2 (1966): 204.

Vogel, M. J. Correspondence. *Canadian Medical Association Journal* 108 (1973): 959.

Vogel, M. J., D. M. Broverman, J. G. Diaguns, and E. L. Klaiber. "The Role of Glutamic Acid in Cognitive Behaviors." *Psychological Bulletin* 65 (1966): 378.

Von Hilsheimer, G. "A Point of View for Teachers and Parents of Special Children Regarding Vitamins and Orthomolecular Medicine." Address presented to Texas Association for Children with Learning Disabilities, Dallas, 1971.

Von Hilsheimer, G., S. D. Klotz, G. McFall, H. Lerner, A. Van West, and D. Quirk. "The Use of Megavitamin Therapy in Regulating Severe Behavior Disorders, Drug Abuse and Frank Psychoses." *Journal of Schizophrenia* 3 (1967): 1.

Watson, G. "Differences in Intermediary Metabolism in Mental Illness." *Psychological Reports* 17 (1965): 563.

———. *Nutrition and Your Mind: The Psychochemical Response.* New York: Harper & Row, 1972.

Watson, G. and W. D. Curier. "Intensive Vitamin Therapy in Mental Illness." *Journal of Psychology* 49 (1960): 67.

Wendel, O. W., and W. E. Beebe. "Preliminary Observations of Altered Carbohydrate Metabolism in Psychiatric Patients." In *Orthomolecular Psychiatry, Treatment of Schizophrenia*, edited by D. Hawkins and L. Pauling. San Francisco: Freeman, 1973.

Wender, P. "Some Speculations Concerning a Possible Biochemical Basis of Minimal Brain Dysfunction." *Annals of the New York Academy of Science* 205 (1973): 21.

Williams, R. J. *Biochemical Individuality.* New York: Wiley, 1957.

———. *Nutrition Against Disease.* New York: Pitman, 1971.

Wohl, M. G. and R. S. Goodhart. *Modern Nutrition in Health and Disease.* Philadelphia: Lea and Febiger, 1968.

Wormsley, G. H. and J. H. Darragh. "Potassium and Sodium Restrictions in the Normal Human." *Journal of Clinical Investigation.* 34 (1955): 456.

Yaryura-Tobias, J. A. "Levodope and Mental Illness." In *Orthomolecular Psychiatry, Treatment of Schizophrenia*, edited by D. Hawkins and L. Pauling. San Francisco: Freeman, 1973.

Yudkin, J. "Myocardial Infarction and Other Diseases of Civilization." *Lancet* 1 (1963): 1335.

Zimmerman, F. T. and S. Ross. "Effect of Glutamic Acid and Other Amino Acids on Maze Learning in the White Rat." *Archives of Neurological Psychiatry* 51 (1944): 446.

SUGGESTED READING FOR PHYSICIANS

Alvarez, W. C. *The Neuroses, Diagnosis and Management of Functional Disorders and Minor Psychoses.* Philadelphia: Saunders, 1952, p. 466.

Amkraut, A., G. F. Solomon, M. Allansmith, B. McClellan, and M. Rappaport. *Archives of General Psychiatry* 28 (May 1973): 673–77.

Arneson, G. A. "Phenothiazine Derivatives and Glucose Metabolism." *Journal of Neuropsychiatry* 5 (1964): 181–85.

Axelrod, A. E. "Nutrition in Relation to Acquired Immunity." In *Modern Nutrition in Health and Disease,* edited by R. S. Goodhart and M. E. Shild. Philadelphia: Lea & Feibiger, 1973.

Axelrod, A. E. and A. C. Traketellis. "Relationship of Pyridoxine to Immunological Phenomena." *Vitamins & Hormones* 22 (1964): 591.

Baird, K. A. *The Human Body and Bacteria: A Study of their Actions and Reactions.* New Brunswick: Bruce Publishing, 1968.

Baker, S. "Fatigue in School Children." *Education Review* 15 (1898): 34.

Bassoe, P. "The Auriculatemporal Syndrome and Other Vasomotor Disturbances About the Head: Auriculatemporal Syndrome Complicating Diseases of Parotid Gland; Angioneuronic Edema of Brain." *Medical Clinics of North America* 16 (1932): 405.

Bell, Iris R. "The Kinin Peptide Hormone Theory of Adaptation and Maladaptation in Psychobiological Illness." Ph.D. dissertation, Stanford University, 1974.

———. "A Kinin Model of Mediation for Food and Chemical Sensitivities: Biobehavioral Implications." *Annals of Allergy* 35 (1975): 206–15.

Berlyne, D. E. *The Reward-Value of Indifferent Stimulation: Reinforcement and Behavior.* New York: Academic Press, 1969, pp. 178–214.

Beyerholm, O. "Gastro-Intestinale Forstyrrelser Ved Dementiapraecox." *Hospitalstidende* 72 (1929): 193.

Bottazzo, G., et al. "Islet-Cell Antibodies in Diabetes Mellitus with Auto-Immune Polyendocrine Deficiencies." *Lancet* 2 (1974): 1279–83.

Brambilla, F., A. Guerrini, F. Riggi, C. Rovere, A. Zanoboni, and W. Zanoboni-Muciaccia. "Glucose-Insulin Metabolism in Chronic Schizophrenia." *Diseases of the Nervous System* 37 (February 1976): 2.

Burton, R. In *The Anatomy of Melancholy,* edited by F. Dell and P. Jordan-Smith. New York: Tudor, 1955, p. 1621.

Buscaino, V. M. "Patologia Extraneurale Della Schizofrenia." *Acta Neurologica* 8 (1958): 1.

Buyze, G., W. J. H. Dries, A. J. Schakelaar, and W. R. P. Schreurs. "The Beneficial Effect of Multiple Vitamin Administration to Psychiatric Patients," in Report of First World Congress of Biological Psychiatry (ler. Congreso Mundial de Psiquiatria Biologiva). Buenos Aires, Argentine Republic, 1974.

Campbell, M. B. "Neurological Allergy." *Review of Allergy* 22 (1968).

———. "Allergy and Behavior: Neurologic and Psychic Syndromes." In *Allergy of the Nervous System,* edited by F. Speer. Springfield, Ill.: Thomas, 1970, pp. 28–46.

———. "Allergy and Epilepsy." In *Allergy of the Nervous System,* edited by F. Speer. Springfield, Ill.: Thomas, 1970.

———. "Neurological Manifestations of Allergic Disease." *Annals of Allergy* 31 (1973).

———. "Neurological and Psychiatric Aspects of Allergy." *The Otolaringologic Clinics of North America: Allergy in Otolaryngologic Practice* 7 (October 1974): 3.

Carlton, P. L. *Brain-Acetylcholine and Inhibition: Reinforcement and Behavior.* New York: Academy Press, 1969.

Carwin, A. H. "The Rotating Diet and Taxonomy." In *Clinical Ecology*, edited by L. Dickey. Springfield, Ill.: Thomas, 1976, pp. 472–86.

Chapman, G. H. Personal Communication to Albert Laverne, editor of *Behavioral Neuropsychiatry*, July 21, 1961.

———. "Microbial Origin of the Gummy Substance of Fujita and Ging." *Transcript of the New York Academy of Sciences II* 25, no. 1 (1962): 66–69.

Cheraskin, E., W. M. Ringsdorg, and J. W. Clark. *Diet and Disease*. Los Angeles: Keats, 1968.

Cleave, T. L. *The Saccharine Disease*. Los Angeles: Keats, 1975.

Coca, A. F. *Familial Nonreagenic Food Allergy*. 3d ed. Springfield, Ill.: Thomas, 1953.

———. *The Pulse Test*. New York: Arco, 1956.

Cooper, K. H. *Aerobics*. New York: Bantam Books, 1969.

Cooper, M. and K. H. Cooper. *Aerobics for Women*. New York: Bantam Books, 1977.

Crook, W. G. "Allergy . . . the Great Masquerader." *Pediatric Basics* (1973).

Dean, G. *The Porphyrias: A Story of Inheritance and Environment*. Philadelphia: Lippincott, 1971.

Dees, S. C. In *Allergy in Relation to Pediatrics*, edited by B. Ratnu. St. Paul & Minneapolis: Bruce, 1951.

Dematteis, F., B. E. Prior, and C. Rimongton. *Nature* 191 (1961): 363.

Dickey, L. D. *Clinical Ecology*. Springfield, Ill.: Thomas, 1976.

Dohan, F. C. and J. C. Grassberger. "Relapsed Schizophrenics: Earlier Discharge from the Hospital After Cereal-Free, Milk-Free Diet." *American Journal of Psychology* 130 (1973): 6.

Dohan, F. C., L. Martin, J. D. Grasberger, D. Boehme, and J. C. Cottrell. "Antibodies to Wheat Gleadin in Blood of Psychiatric Patients: Possible Role of Emotional Factors." *Biological Psychiatry* 5, no. 2 (1972): 127–37.

Dolowitz, D. A. "Drug Treatment in Allergic Disorders." *The Otolaryngologic Clinics of North America: Allergy in Otolaryngologic Practice* (1971): 598.

Eastham, R. D. *Biochemical Values in Clinical Medicine.* Baltimore: Williams & Wilkins, 1971.

Ellis, J. *Vitamin B_6, The Doctor's Report.* New York: Harper & Row, 1973.

Fishman, M. "Brain Stem Lesions in Schizophrenia." *Roche Report: Frontiers of Psychiatry* 3 (1976).

———. "Encephalitic Lesions Found in Brains of Schizophrenics." *Clinical Psychiatry News* (December 1977): 3.

Fleischman, A. I., W. H. Philpott, G. Van Hilscheimer, L. Moore, P. N. Milner, and S. C. Klatz. "Lipid Chemistry and the Psychiatric Patient." *Journal of Orthomolecular Psychiatry* 4, no. 2 (1975): 168–73.

Franzen, G. *Psychiatric Clinic* 5 (1972): 201–8.

Frier, B. M., et al. "Exocrine Pancreatic Function in Juvenile-Onset Diabetes Mellitus." *Gut* 17 (1976): 685–91.

Fuller, H. L. "Sublingual Heparin in Hyperglycemia: A Preliminary Report." *Angiology* (1958): 311.

———. "Effect of Sublingual Heparin on Lypemia Clearing and on Recurrence of Myocardial Infarction." *Angiology* (1960): 200.

Furlong, F. W. *Canadian Psychiatric Association Journal* 20 (December 1975): 577–83.

Galtman, A. M. "Mechanism of Migraine." *Journal of Allergy* 7 (1936): 351.

Gambill, E. E. *Pancreatitis.* St. Louis. Mo.: Mosby, 1973.

Goldberg, A. *Porphyrins and Porphyrias in Recent Advances in Hematology.* Edinburgh: Churchill Livingstone, 1971.

Goodman, L. S. and A. Gilman. *The Pharmacological Basis of Therapeutics.* New York: Macmillan, 1970.

Greden, J. F. "Anxiety or Caffeinism: A Diagnostic Dilemma." *American Journal of Psychiatry* 13, no. 10 (October 1974): 1089–92.

Guyton, A. C. *Textbook of Medical Physiology.* 4th ed. Philadelphia: Saunders, 1971.

Harper, H. A. *Review of Physiological Chemistry.* 10th ed. Los Altos, Calif.: Lange, 1965, p. 240.

Harvey, A. M., R. J. Johns, A. H. Owens, and R. S. Ross, eds. *The Principles and Practice of Medicine.* New York: Appleton-Century-Crofts, 1972, p. 879.

Hearst, E. "The Effects of Scopolamine on Discriminated Responding in the Rat." *Journal of Pharmacology and Experimental Therapeutics,* 1959.

Hiles, B. W. "Hyperglycemia and Glycasuria Following Cholorpromazine Therapy." *Journal of the American Medical Association* 162 (1956): 165.

Hoffer, A. "Senility and Chronic Malnutrition." *Journal of Orthomolecular Psychiatry* 3, no. 1 (1974).

Hoffer, A. and H. Osmond. *How to Live with Schizophrenia.* New Hyde Park, N.Y.: University Books, 1966.

Jordan, D. R. *Dyslexia in the Classroom.* Columbus, Ohio: Merrill, 1972.

Kalokerinos, A. *Every Second Child.* Australia: Thomas Nelson, 1974.

Kellermeyer, R. W. and R. C. Graham. "Kinnis: Possible Physiologic and Pathologic Role in Man." *New England Journal of Medicine* 279 (1962): 859.

Klenner, F. R. "Observations on the Dose and Administration of Ascorbic Acid When Employed Beyond the Range of a Vitamin in Human Pathology." *Journal of Applied Nutrition* 23 (1971): 61.

Kolb, L. D. *Noyes' Modern Clinical Psychiatry.* Philadelphia: Saunders, 1968.

Lee, J. B. *The Prostaglandins Textbook of Endocrinology.* Philadelphia: Saunders, 1974.

Lehman, H. E. "Schizophrenia IV: Clinical Features." In *Comprehensive Textbook of Psychiatry,* edited by A. M. Freedman and H. Kaplan. Baltimore: Williams & Wilkins, 1967, p. 128.

Levine, S. *Hormones and Conditioning.* Nebraska: University of Nebraska Press, 1968.

Livingston, A. M., V. Wuerthele-Caspe Livingston, E. Alexander-Jackson, and G. H. Wolter. "Toxic Fractions Obtained from Tumor

Isolates and Related Clinical Implications." *Annals of the New York Academy of Sciences* 174, no. 2 (October 1970): 675–89.

Livingston, V. and E. Alexander-Jackson. "A Specific Type of Organism Cultivated from Malignancy: Bacteriology and Proposed Classification." *Annals of the New York Academy of Sciences* 174 (1970): 2.

Livingston, V. Wuerthele-Caspe and A. M. Livingston. "Demonstration of Progenitor Cryptocides in the Blood of Patients with Collagen and Neoplastic Diseases." *Transcript of the New York Academy of Sciences* 34, no. 5 (January 1972): 433–53.

———. "Some Cultural, Immunological and Biochemical Properties of Progenitor Cryptocides." *Transcript of the New York Academy of Sciences* 36, no. 6 (June 1974): 569–82.

MacCuish, A., et al. "Antibodies to Pancreatic Islet Cells in Insulin-Dependent Diabetics with Coexistent Autoimmune Disease." *Lancet* 7896 (December 28, 1976): 1529–31.

Mandell, M. *Cerebral Reactions in Allergic Patients.* New England Foundation for Allergic and Environmental Disease, Norwalk, Connecticut, 1969.

———. "Central Nervous System Hypersensitivity to House Dust, Molds, and Foods." *Review of Allergy* 24 (1970): 4.

———. "Ecologic Allergic and Metabolic Factors in the Etiology of Physical and Mental Disorders." *New Dynamics of Preventive Medicine.* New York: Intercontinental, 1974.

McGovern, J. D. and T. J. Hayward. *Allergic Headache: Allergy of the Nervous System.* Springfield, Ill.: Thomas, 1970, pp. 47–58.

Meyer, Fr. "Anatomisch-histologische untersuchungen an schizophrenen." *Monatschr f. Psychiat. u. Nurol.* 91 (1935): 185.

Miller, J. B. *Food Allergy, Provocative Testing and Injection Therapy.* Springfield, Ill.: Thomas.

Moyer, K. E. "The Physiology of Violence: Allergy and Aggression." *Psychology Today* (July 1975).

Newbold, H. L. "Autogenous Urine Therapy" (personal communication). 251 East 51st St., New York, NY 10022, 1974.

Norman, D. and W. A. Hiestrand. "Glycemic Effects of Chlorpromazine in the Mouse, Hamster and Rat. *Proceedings of the Society for Experimental Biology and Medicine* 90 (1955): 89–91.

Ostfield, A., L. F. Chapman, H. Goodell, and H. G. Wolff. "Studies in Headache; Summary of Evidence Concerning Noxious Agents Active Locally During Migraine Headache." *Psychosomatic Medicine* 19 (1957): 199.

Papez, J. W. "Inclusion Bodies Associated with Destruction of Nerve Cells in Scrub Typhus, Psychoses and Multiple Sclerosis." *Journal of Nervous and Mental Disease* 108 (1948): 5.

———. "A Study of Polyzoan Organisms in Brains of Young and Mentally Ill Patients." *Journal of Gerontology* 7 (1952): 3.

———. "Demonstrations—Living Organisms in Nerve Cells as Seen Under Dark Contrast Phase Microscope." *Transcript of the American Neurological Association*, 1952.

———. "Form of Living Organisms in Psychotic Patients." *Journal of Nervous and Mental Disease* 116 (1952): 5.

Papez, J. W. and B. Pearl Papez. "The Hypophysis Crebri in Psychosis." *Journal of Nervous and Mental Disease* 119 (1954): 4.

———. "Drops of Protein in Brains of Hospital Patients in Stupor, Uremia, Edema, Clouded, and Catatonic States." *Journal of Nervous and Mental Disease* 12 (1956): 4.

———. "Arteriolar Mycosis Associated with Chronic Degenerative Brain Disease (A New Look at Sclerotic Patches)." *Diseases of the Nervous System* 16 (1957): 4.

Papez, J. W. and J. F. Bateman. "Cytological Changes in Cells of Thalmic Nuclei in Senile, Paranoid and Manic Psychoses." *Journal of Nervous and Mental Disease* 112 (1950): 5.

———. "Changes in Nervous Tissues and Study of Living Organisms in Mental Disease." *Journal of Nervous and Mental Disease* 114 (1951): 5.

Passwater, R. *Selenium as Food and Medicine*. Los Angeles: Keats, 1980.

Pauling, L. "Orthomolecular Psychiatry." *Scientific Journal* 160 (1968): 265–71.

Perry, T. L., S. Hansen, B. Tischlet, F. M. Richards, and M. Sokol. "Unrecognized Adult Phenylketonuria: Implications for Obstetrics and Psychiatry." *New England Journal of Medicine* 298 (1973): 8.

Peters, H. A. "Trace Minerals, Chelating Agents and the Porphyrias." *Federal Proceedings* 20 (1971): 3.

Peters, H. A., P. L. Eichman, and H. H. Reese. "Therapy of Acute, Chronic and Mixed Hepatic Porphyria Patients with Chelating Agents." *Neurology* 8 (1958): 8.

Peters, H. A., S. A. M. Johnson, S. Cam, S. Oral, Y. Muftu, and T. Ergene. "Hexachlorobenzene-Induced Porphyria: Effect of Chelation on the Disease, Porphyrin and Metal Metabolism." *American Journal of Medical Sciences* 251 (1966): 3.

Peters, H. A., S. Woods, P. L. Eichman, and H. H. Reese. "The Treatment of Acute Porphyria with Chelating Agents: A Report of 21 Cases." *Annals of Internal Medicine* 47 (1957): 5.

Pfeiffer, C. C. *Mental and Elemental Nutrients.* Los Angeles: Keats, 1975, p. 419.

Philpott, W. H. "Chemical Defects, Allergic and Toxic States as Causes and/or Facilitating Factors of Emotional Reactions, Dyslexia, Hyperkinesis, and Learning Problems." *Journal of the International Academy of Metabology* 2 (1973): 58.

———. "Sedac Treatment, Post Sedac, Response Interference and Electric Shock." *Diseases of the Nervous System* 34 (1973): 2.

———. "Maladaptive Reactions to Frequently Used Foods and Commonly Met Chemicals as Precipitating Factors in Many Chronic Physical and Chronic Emotional Illnesses." *New Dynamics of Preventive Medicine.* New York: Intercontinental, 1974.

———. "Methods of Relief of Acute and Chronic Symptoms of Deficiency-Allergy-Addiction Maladaptive Reactions to Foods and Chemicals." In *Clinical Ecology,* edited by L. D. Dickey. Springfield, Ill.: Thomas, 1976, pp. 496–509.

———. "Ecologic and Biochemical Observations in the Schizophrenic Syndrome." *Journal of Orthomolecular Psychiatry* 6 (1977): 277–82.

———. "Professional Dyslexia About Dyslexia." *Journal of Orthomolecular Psychiatry* 6 (1977): 27–32.

———. "The Role of Allergy-Addiction in the Disease Process." *New Dynamics of Preventive Medicine* 5 (1977): 99–104.

Philpott, W. H., R. Neilsen, and V. Pearson. "Four-Day Rotation of Foods According to Families." In *Clinical Ecology,* edited by L. D. Dickey. Springfield. Ill.: Thomas, 1976, pp. 472–86.

Potts, J. and M. S. Lang. "Avoidance Provocative Food Testing in Assessing Diabetes Responsiveness." *Diabetes* 26 (1977).

Randolph, T. G. "Food Allergy and Food Addiction." 9th Annual Congress, American College of Allergists, Chicago, 1953.

———. "The Specific Adaptation Syndrome." *Journal of Laboratory and Clinical Medicine* 48 (1956): 934 (abstract).

———. "Ecologic Mental Illness—Levels of Central Nervous System Reactions." *Proceedings of Third World Congress of Psychiatry*. Montreal, Canada: University of Toronto Press, June 1961, pp. 379–84.

———. "The Ecologic Unit, Part 1 and Part 11." *Hospital Management,* March and April, 1964.

———. "Ecologically Oriented Medicine: Its Need, I. Comparison with Anthropocentric Medicine, II. The Roles of Specific Adaptation and Individual Susceptibility in Chronic Illness, III. Stimulatory and Withdrawal Manifestations of Specific Reactions, IV." 1973. Human Ecology Research Organization, 50 North Lake Shore Drive, Chicago, IL 60611.

———. "The History of Ecologic Mental Illness." In *Annual Review of Allergy,* edited by C. A. Frazier, 1973, pp. 425–41. Flushing, N.Y: Medical Examination Publishing, 1974.

———. "Adaptation to Specific Environmental Exposures Enhanced by Individual Susceptibility." In *Clinical Ecology,* edited by L. D. Dickey. Springfield, Ill.: Thomas, 1976, pp. 45–66.

———. "Biological Dietetics." In *Clinical Ecology,* edited by L. D. Dickey. Springfield, Ill.: Thomas, 1976, pp. 107–21.

———. "The Enzymatic, Acid, Pypoxia, Endocrine Concept of Allergic Inflammation." In *Clinical Ecology,* edited by L. D. Dickey. Springfield, Ill.: Thomas, 1976, pp. 577–96.

———. "Hospital Comprehensive Environmental Control Program." In *Clinical Ecology,* edited by L. D. Dickey. Springfield, Ill.: Thomas, 1976, pp. 70–85.

Randolph, T. G. and J. P. Rollins. "Beet Sensitivity: Allergic Reactions from Ingestion of Beet Sugar (Sucrose) and Monosodium Glutamate of Beef Origin." *Journal of Laboratory and Clinical Medicine* 36 (September 1950): 407–15.

Rapaport, H. G. and S. H. Flint. "Is There a Relationship Between Allergy and Learning Disabilities?" *Journal of School Health* 46, no. 3 (March 1976).

Rapaport, H. G. and S. M. Linde. *The Complete Allergy Guide.* New York: Simon and Schuster, 1970.

Reich, C. J. "The Vitamin Therapy of Chronic Asthma." *Journal of Asthma Research* 9 (1971): 32.

Reiter, P. J. *Zur pathologie der dementia praecox-gastrointestinale storungen. Ihre klinische und aetologische bedeutung.* Leipzig: George Thiemes Verlag, 1929.

Richet, C. "Anaphylaxis in General and Anaphylaxis to Mytilocongestine in Particular." *Annals of the Institute of Pasteur* 21 (1907): 497.

Rinkel, H. J., T. G. Randolph, and M. Zeller. *Food Allergy.* Springfield, Ill.: Thomas, 1951.

Rowe, A. H. *Elimination Diets and the Patient's Allergies.* Philadelphia: Lea and Febiger, 1944.

———. "Clinical Allergy in the Nervous System." *Quarterly Review of Allergy Applied Immunology* 6 (1952): 157.

Rowe, A. H. and A. Rowe, Jr. *Food Allergy (Its Manifestations and Control and the Elimination Diets): A Compendium.* Springfield, Ill.: Thomas, 1972.

Selye, H. *Textbook of Endocrinology.* 1st ed. Montreal: Acta Endocrinologica, Université de Montreal, 1947, p. 914.

———. *The Stress of Life.* New York: McGraw-Hill, 1956.

———. *Stress Without Distress.* New York: Lippincott, 1974.

———. *Stress in Health and Disease.* Boston: Butterworth Publishers, 1976, p.1256.

Silva, R. E. and G. Kasmin, eds. *Polypeptidase and Biogenic Amines in Acute Inflammatory Reactions: Endocrinic Aspects of Disease.* St. Louis, Mo.: Warren H. Green, 1968.

Singh, M. and S. R. Kay. *Science* 191 (January 30, 1976): 401–2.

Speer, F. *Allergy of the Nervous System.* Springfield, Ill.: Thomas, 1970.

Spies, T. D. "The Response of Pellagrins to Nicotonic Acid." *Lancet* (January 29, 1938).

Spies, T. D., W. B. Bean, and R. E. Stone. "The Treatment of Subclinical and Classic Pellagra." *Journal of the American Medical Association* (1938).

Stone, I. *The Healing Factor, "Vitamin C" Against Disease.* New York: Gosset & Dunlap, 1972.

Thonnard, N. E. "Phenothiazines and Diabetes in Hospitalized Women." *American Journal of Psychiatry* 124 (1968): 978–82.

Tintera, J. W. "The Hypoadrenocortical State and Its Management." *New York State Journal of Medicine* 55 (1955): 1869.

———. "Stabilizing Homeostasis in the Recovered Alcoholic Through Endocrine Therapy: Evaluation of the Hypoglycemia Factor." *Journal of the American Geriatric Society* 14 (1966): 126.

———. "Endocrine Aspects of Schizophrenia: Hypoglycemia of Hypoadrenocorticism." *Journal of Schizophrenia* 1 (1967): 150.

Torrey, E. F. and M. Peterson. "Slow and Latent Viruses in Schizophrenia." *Lancet* 2 (1973): 22.

Torrey, E. F., B. B. Torrey, and B. G. Burton-Bradley. "The Epidemiology of Schizophrenia in Papua New Guinea." *American Journal of Psychiatry* 131 (May 1974): 5.

Waitzkin, L. "A Survey of Unknown Diabetics in a Mental Hospital." *Diabetes* 15 (1966): 97–104.

Watson, G. *Nutrition and Your Mind.* New York: Harper & Row, 1972.

Weiss, J. M. and H. S. Kaufman. "A Subtle Organic Component in Some Cases of Mental Illness." *Archives of General Psychiatry* 25 (July 1971).

Williams, R. *Nutrition Against Disease: Environmental Prevention.* New York: Pitman, 1971.

Williams, R. J. and D. A. Kalita. *A Physician's Handbook on Orthomolecular Medicine.* Los Angeles: Keats, 1979, p. 78.

Wolf, M. and K. Ransberger. *Enzyme Therapy.* Los Angeles: Regent House, 1972.

Zumoff, B. and L. Helman. "Aggravation of Diabetic Hyperglycemia by Chlacodiazephoxide." *Journal of the American Medical Association* 237 (1977): 18.

INDEX

('i' indicates an illustration, 't' indicates a table)

O

P

U

V

W-Y-Z